Cambridge Elements ≡

Elements of Improving Quality and Safety in Healthcare
edited by
Mary Dixon-Woods,* Katrina Brown,* Sonja Marjanovic,†
Tom Ling,† Ellen Perry,* and Graham Martin*
*THIS Institute (The Healthcare Improvement Studies Institute)
†RAND Europe

WORKPLACE CONDITIONS

Jill Maben,[1] Jane Ball,[2] and
Amy C. Edmondson[3]

[1]School of Health Sciences, University of Surrey
[2]School of Health Sciences, University of Southampton
[3]Harvard Business School

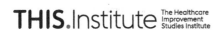
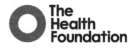

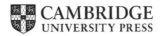

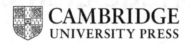

CAMBRIDGE
UNIVERSITY PRESS

Shaftesbury Road, Cambridge CB2 8EA, United Kingdom

One Liberty Plaza, 20th Floor, New York, NY 10006, USA

477 Williamstown Road, Port Melbourne, VIC 3207, Australia

314–321, 3rd Floor, Plot 3, Splendor Forum, Jasola District Centre,
New Delhi – 110025, India

103 Penang Road, #05–06/07, Visioncrest Commercial, Singapore 238467

Cambridge University Press is part of Cambridge University Press & Assessment,
a department of the University of Cambridge.

We share the University's mission to contribute to society through the pursuit of
education, learning and research at the highest international levels of excellence.

www.cambridge.org
Information on this title: www.cambridge.org/9781009363860

DOI: 10.1017/9781009363839

First published 2023

A catalogue record for this publication is available from the British Library.

ISBN 978-1-009-36386-0 Paperback
ISSN 2754-2912 (online)
ISSN 2754-2904 (print)

Workplace Conditions

Elements of Improving Quality and Safety in Healthcare

DOI: 10.1017/9781009363839
First published online: January 2023

Jill Maben,[1] Jane Ball,[2] and Amy C. Edmondson[3]
[1]School of Health Sciences, University of Surrey
[2]School of Health Sciences, University of Southampton
[3]Harvard Business School

Author for correspondence: Jill Maben, j.maben@surrey.ac.uk

Abstract: This Element reviews the evidence for three workplace conditions that matter for improving quality and safety in healthcare: staffing; psychological safety, teamwork, and speaking up; and staff health and well-being at work. The authors propose that these are environmental prerequisites for improvement. They examine how staff numbers and skills are related to the quality of care provided and the ability to improve it. They present evidence for the importance of psychological safety, teamwork, and speaking up, noting that these are interrelated and critical for healthcare improvement. They present evidence of associations between staff well-being at work and patient outcomes. Finally, they suggest healthcare improvement should be embedded into the day-to-day work of frontline staff; adequate time and resources must be provided, with quality as the mainstay of professionals' work. Every day at every level, the working context must support the question, 'how could we do this better?' This title is also available as Open Access on Cambridge Core.

Keywords: workplace conditions, nurse staffing, psychological safety, healthcare teams, staff well-being

ISBNs: 9781009363860 (PB), 9781009363839 (OC)
ISSNs: 2754-2912 (online), 2754-2904 (print)

Contents

1 Introduction

This Element examines the workplace conditions that underpin successful improvement of quality and safety in healthcare. It highlights aspects of the workforce and working environment that may thwart or support healthcare improvement in practice, while recognising that good workplace conditions can also be *outcomes* of healthcare improvement. We examine the role of three key workplace conditions that are prerequisites for the work of improving quality and safety in healthcare: staffing for quality; psychological safety, teamwork and speaking up; and staff health and well-being at work. We summarise the evidence and show how each contributes to organisational capacity to deliver quality and safety and enable improvement, and explain how success can be assessed.

There may be little dispute about some of the preconditions (funding, staffing, training) for improving quality and safety. But many of the issues we present in this Element operate at multiple levels and vary within and between organisations and workplace units, since staff experiences are shaped by their immediate teams as well as the whole organisational context and culture. Accordingly, much of our analysis is based on the principle that, fundamentally, healthcare work is interactional. People's actions, interactions, and relationships with each other are critical to enabling an organisation to adopt, implement, and sustain improvements.

2 Staffing for Quality

Staffing (including numbers and skills) can be seen as a structural prerequisite – in Donabedian's sense of structure[1] – both for providing high-quality, safe care and for improving care. A large body of evidence suggests that having the right numbers of staff and skills affects patient care quality and patient outcomes, as well as staff well-being and engagement, staff absence sickness rates, retention, and burnout.[2–6] The links between staff well-being at work and patient experience are also well established[7,8] (this is discussed in more detail in Section 4).

Most evidence on staffing relates specifically to nurses and is therefore a key focus of this Element. Much less common is research examining staffing from a whole-team perspective or looking at the impact of staffing levels in other groups (e.g. medical, pharmacy, administrative, and facilities staff[9–11]) on quality or patient outcomes. However, much learning from the staffing literature on nursing may be generalisable, particularly given the key role of nurses in driving the quality of care and improvement in many settings.[12,13] In this section, we present an overview of the research evidence on links between nurse staffing and quality in acute hospitals; consider the concept of staffing sufficiency and how it is translated into policies and guidance; look at how nurse staffing is applied in practice in relation to quality; and consider the role of nursing staff in improving care quality.

2.1 Staffing and Care Quality: The Evidence Base

A striking finding of decades of research, covering hundreds of studies systematically reviewed on multiple occasions,[2,14,15] is the association between registered nurse staffing, care quality, and patient outcomes. Lower registered nurse staffing is associated with poorer care quality and worse outcomes for patients. This is evident, for example, in the finding of a significant effect of both medical and nurse staffing levels in intensive care units in England on casemix-adjusted patient mortality.[11] Both the total volume of nursing hours (as captured by ratios or by measures such as nursing hours per patient day) and the proportion of the nursing workforce that is degree-educated (as opposed to assistants and support workers without formal qualifications or registration) are important to care quality.[16,17] The evidence base on the relationship between nurse staffing and care quality is heavily biased towards studies in general acute hospitals, but a number of key studies cover other settings, such as mental health,[18,19] nursing homes,[20] and primary care.[21,22]

A 2006 systematic review of 101 studies confirmed a relationship between low levels of registered nurse staffing and adverse patient outcomes, with a meta-analysis of data from 28 of those studies finding that higher nurse staffing was associated with lower odds of hospital-related mortality and adverse patient events.[2] More recently, a 2014 review of evidence (including systematic reviews) for the National Institute for Health and Care Excellence (NICE) – to support development of guidelines for safe nurse staffing in adult inpatient acute settings in England – identified 35 primary studies since 2006 looking at nurse staffing and patient outcomes.[23] A summary of findings is set out in Box 1.[24]

The pattern of findings is broadly consistent across the substantial evidence base: when levels of registered nurse staffing are lower, outcomes are poorer. Analysis of data from nine European countries in the RN4CAST study, for example, found that an increase in a nurse's workload by one patient is associated with a 7% increased likelihood of patient death following common types of surgery;[25] and the mix of nursing staff (proportion of registered nurses vs care assistants) and their education levels (proportion of workforce that is degree educated) is associated with differences in patient outcomes and experiences.[16,17]

2.1.1 The Plausibility of a Causal Link

Though the causal relationship between nurse staffing and patient outcomes may seem probable, there are limitations in the research.[15] One key weakness is

Box 1 SUMMARY OF FINDINGS FROM 2014 EVIDENCE REVIEW FOR NICE

- Strong evidence from several large observational studies that lower nurse staffing levels were associated with higher rates of death and falls.
- Strong evidence that higher nurse staffing is associated with reduced length of stay and lower readmission rates.
- Similar but less consistent evidence on infections.
- Contradictory evidence on pressure ulcers.
- No evidence of an association with venous thromboembolism.

Reproduced from Ball and Griffiths,[24] in accordance with the terms of the Creative Commons licence (http://creativecommons.org/licenses/by/4.0)

that most studies have a cross-sectional (one-off) design, rather than a longitudinal (over time) design. However, research evidence increasingly suggests not only that low staffing is *associated* with worse outcomes, but that the relationship with care outcomes is *causal*.[26–28] In 2011, Needleman et al. broke the mould in nursing workforce and patient outcome research with a US longitudinal study that looked at individual patient outcomes following exposure to low nurse staffing.[28] Using administrative data to capture nurse staffing for every shift, a significantly increased risk of mortality (taking account of patient factors) was observed *after* periods of exposure to low staffing.

Other research also supports the plausibility of a causal link between staffing, care quality, and patient outcomes. When nurse staffing levels are lower, there is an increased risk of necessary patient care being missed.[17,29] This is a simple but highly significant finding, considering how staffing levels affect services' ability to achieve (and improve) care quality. Nine out of 10 nurses on acute wards in 32 National Health Service (NHS) hospital trusts reported having left at least one aspect of care (i.e. that was needed by their patients) 'undone' on their last shift due to lack of time. The amount of care left undone was strongly related to nurses' reports on the quality of nursing care on the ward and their ratings of the ward's environment for patient safety.[29]

Further analysis of data from the RN4CAST study[30] points to 'missed nursing care' as partially mediating the relationship between nurse staffing and avoidable patient mortality.[17,29,31] Taking account of different risk factors (e.g. patient age and health conditions), more patients die following common surgical procedures when levels of missed care reported by nurses are higher; an additional 10% of missed care was associated with a 16% increased risk of patient death.[31]

Findings from a retrospective longitudinal observational study in the NHS confirm the pattern identified by Needleman et al.[28] and indicated by the RN4CAST analyses. Using routinely collected staffing data over a 3-year period, the study examined its relationship with casemix-adjusted patient mortality.[27,32] The hazard of death increased by 3% for every day that a patient experienced nurse staffing that fell below the average for that ward.[32,33]

This more recent evidence supports a plausible causal link between nurse staffing levels and patient outcomes. It points to the idea that the number of registered nurses present to provide care influences the ability of a team (potentially beyond the immediate nursing team) to deliver care completely. Nurse staffing sufficiency is thus key to reducing negative care incidents associated with low staffing – such as errors, adverse events, and omissions – which may contribute to potentially avoidable deaths in some cases.[34,35]

2.1.2 How Many Is Enough?

Despite the strength of the evidence to support the general association between nurse staffing and patient outcomes, studies offer little specificity about exactly *what* level of nurse staffing is required to enable good quality care to flourish – that is, how many is enough? Few studies go beyond establishing a statistically significant association to provide detailed information on the numbers associated with different effects.

A US study showed that a significant increase in mortality was associated with patients' exposure to nurse 'short-staffing' (defined as 8 or more nursing hours per shift below the target staffing level identified using a validated staffing tool).[28] And NICE guidance for NHS hospitals identifies a daytime threshold of more than eight adult patients per registered nurse on an acute ward as associated with increased risk.[36] (Of course, this varies according to the ward or unit, and for some services significant increases in risk occur well below this threshold.) The guidance does not specify what constitutes a safe minimum but does provide an indication of what unsafe might look like. NICE's interpretation of the evidence is that a ratio of one nurse to eight patients is not likely to represent an optimal safe-staffing level in any setting; rather, it is a level at which risk is known to increase and therefore a threshold that demands urgent review.

Evidence from the NHS is consistent with international research showing that lower nurse staffing levels are associated with worse outcomes in a variety of acute ward contexts. But an outstanding question concerns the nature of the relationship between staffing and outcomes: is it a standard performance curve in which the benefits of greater nurse staffing gradually taper off once an optimal threshold is reached? In an in-depth study in a single NHS hospital trust,[32] we explicitly tested for – and found – a linear relationship between patient-level exposure to staffing at different levels and benefits; but we did not find a threshold effect. Patient benefit increased in direct proportion to increased nursing hours. Although there was a range of staffing levels across the hospital wards, we did not find a beyond optimum level – where the benefit of additional registered nurses starts to plateau.

2.2 Sufficient Staffing: Policies, Regulations, and Guidance

The principle of having sufficient staff (including nursing staff) for safe and effective care is embodied in policies, regulations, and guidance – and, in some parts of the world, in legislation. In the UK, the NHS Constitution states that patients have the 'right to be treated with a professional standard of care, by appropriately qualified and experienced staff, in a properly approved or registered organisation that meets required levels of safety and quality'.[37] From a public safety perspective, the Nursing and Midwifery Council's professional code is explicit about the obligation of staff to raise concerns if staffing levels risk patient safety: '[You must] act without delay if you believe that there is a risk to patient safety or public protection.'[38]

Different approaches are taken to determining safe staffing, with some contention around which is most effective. The pros and cons of mandated minimums have been debated for years.[39] Much of the argument stems from an artificial polarisation of the issue: the idea of mandated minimum ratios versus dependency-based tools to support local decision-making. Arguably, each has a place: a limit to ensure safety standards across a system, and judgement and tools to determine optimum levels in different contexts. But the principle that adequate nurse staffing is required to deliver high-quality care is not in question; throughout the world, it consistently underpins policies, guidance, and sometimes legislation.

In parts of the USA and Australia, the law stipulates a minimum nurse staffing level. The number of open beds and patients is limited by the number of staff present. For example, in California[40] and two Australian states[41] the safe daytime minimum for an acute ward is typically one registered nurse to five patients. Proponents see this as a safety measure that protects staffing levels from becoming dangerously low; opponents see it as too blunt a measure and fear that, in a context of cost constraints and labour market challenges, a minimum can become a maximum.[42]

Policy and law vary within the UK. In Wales and Scotland, legislation is similar to that in many parts of the USA: it makes explicit the principle of ensuring staffing levels are evidence-based, using approved tools or measures to ensure nurse staffing is sufficient to meet patient needs safely. In Northern Ireland, the

Delivering Care framework included normative ranges in addition to guidance to support staffing for high-quality care.[43] But in England, numbers and the proportion of registered nurses within the nursing team (referred to as the 'skill mix') have been determined locally by individual healthcare organisations.

In its role as healthcare regulator, the Care Quality Commission (CQC) ensures compliance with Regulation 18, which requires healthcare providers in England to 'provide sufficient numbers of suitably qualified, competent, skilled and experienced staff to meet the needs of the people using the service at all times'.[44] But the challenge for providers is gauging what is sufficient to enable not just safe but high-quality care. Following the 2013 inquiry into the care crisis at the Mid Staffordshire NHS Foundation Trust,[45] NICE introduced guidance recommending that a daytime level of eight patients or more per registered nurse on acute wards should be considered a 'warning' – triggering an urgent review of metrics and staffing.[36,46]

2.3 Putting Staffing into Practice to Improve Quality

NICE guidelines for safe staffing highlight the need for a robust assessment of the nurse staffing levels required to meet patient needs on acute wards, and endorse a tool (the Safer Nursing Care Tool) for this purpose.[36] But even with an accurate estimation of need and employers willing to increase staffing to ensure sufficient baseline numbers, challenges in recruitment and retention may stymie efforts to achieve those numbers, as has been the case in the NHS.[47] Attention to the wider factors that influence recruitment and retention is therefore key,[48–50] but one of the biggest drivers for nurses leaving the profession is too much pressure (cited second after retirement in the Nursing and Midwifery Council's surveys of leavers).[51] This highlights a degree of circularity at the heart of the issue: having enough staff is key to having enough staff.

The ability of healthcare organisations to employ sufficient numbers of registered nurses to achieve high-quality care depends not only on recognising necessary staffing levels but also on an effective labour market. In a study on the implementation of safe-staffing policies in England, directors of nursing reported that despite board-level commitment to increase nurse staffing, the biggest impediment to achieving the levels needed was an ongoing national shortage of nurses.[47] This is a worldwide challenge, which in the USA led to a specific organisational model: Magnet hospitals.

2.3.1 Magnet Hospitals

In a context of widespread shortages of registered nurses in the USA in the late 1980s, researchers identified considerable differences between hospitals'

Box 2 Characteristics of Magnet hospitals[48,53]

- Flatter organisational structures.
- Good staffing (higher nurse-to-patient ratios).
- Collaborative relationships between nurses and doctors.
- Broad-based participation in decision-making related to clinical care.
- Sufficient core staff (limited use of agency/temporary staffing).
- Nursing research that enhances clinical practice.
- Higher percentage of degree-educated or masters-educated registered nurses.
- Influential nurse executives and visible nursing leadership.
- Investment in the education and expertise of nurses.
- Better retention and lower turnover of registered nurses.
- Positive practice environment with good working conditions.
- Nurses feel well supported (e.g. by support services and availability of resources) to provide high-quality care.

abilities to recruit and retain nurses.[48] Some were struggling. But others were succeeding, as though they had magnetic properties that enabled them to attract and keep their nursing staff. These hospitals also had reputations for good quality patient care – a factor that made them attractive to nurses. The positive attributes that made Magnet hospitals attractive places to work were subsequently found to correlate with better patient outcomes (e.g. lower casemix-adjusted patient mortality rates).[52] Typical characteristics of Magnet hospitals are summarised in Box 2. We include traits that these hospitals tend to have (based on the original research[48]), standards they are expected to have achieved (American Nurses Credentialing Center standards), and characteristics identified in research comparing Magnet and non-Magnet hospitals.[53]

The Magnet phenomenon generated considerable interest in the USA.[54] Research examining the features associated with Magnet hospitals[48,55,56] was crucial in establishing that the relationship between nurse staffing and quality is about more than just numbers: a positive working environment is also critically important. Though some factors that may influence a hospital's ability to keep staff may be intractable (e.g. location, cost of living), many of the characteristics associated with better retention and lower turnover are potentially modifiable (e.g. leadership, communication, and teamwork).

Based on this learning, the American Nurses Association developed a quality improvement programme and established the American Nurses Credentialing

Center to help other centres develop the characteristics to achieve Magnet status. Study of the features of Magnet hospitals since then suggests they are associated with better patient outcomes as well as better work environments.[57–59] Kelly et al. report that Magnet hospitals are more likely to have working environments that are supportive of professional nursing care than other hospitals, and to employ more highly educated nurses. They also found that nurses in Magnet hospitals were less likely to be dissatisfied with their jobs or report high burnout.[53]

In 2020 there were 468 healthcare providers in five countries formally accredited as Magnets, but relatively few outside the USA. Adoption of an English Magnet model was proposed in 2015 in Lord Willis's report on nursing, but there have been mixed views about the usefulness and transferability of the model.[54,60,61] In common with other accreditation schemes, what is unclear is whether the process of *becoming* a Magnet improves quality or whether the high quality and outcomes achieved by Magnets mean that better hospitals are just better.[62] A study launched in 2020 in five European countries, which includes a randomised controlled trial of the intervention and a process evaluation, will allow a more complete examination of the claimed 'transformative effect' of adopting Magnet principles and shed some light on the relative importance of different elements.[63]

Either way, the fact that positive nurse staffing traits (good nurse staffing levels, proportion of the workforce with a degree or a higher degree, visible nursing leadership) go hand in hand with success in achieving quality – or, in Magnet terminology, 'nursing excellence' – is a testament to the importance of these staffing conditions. It seems likely that the relationships between improvement and staffing may operate in the other direction also; improvement work can create better work conditions, leading to less staff stress and improved staff engagement, which may result in a more efficient use of the staff available.

2.3.2 Assessing the Impact of Staffing Changes

Healthcare organisations need some means of assessing whether they have the staffing and work conditions needed for quality and for improvement. Finding feasible and meaningful indicators for the structures, processes, and outcomes is a recognised challenge,[64] but it is essential to improvement. (For further consideration, see the Element on measurement for improvement.[65])

We earlier referred to the important research finding that care left undone is associated with low staffing (Section 2.1.1). In Ireland, this has led to its use as an indicator[66] which was adopted by the government. Care left undone events (referred to as safety CLUEs) were used as a metric to assess signs of insufficiency and measure improvement as staffing levels were increased (Box 3).[66]

> Box 3 PUTTING EVIDENCE INTO PRACTICE: A NURSE STAFFING FRAMEWORK
> TO IMPROVE QUALITY
>
> Objective: to apply an evidence-based approach to nurse staffing in healthcare.
>
> **Key Project Phases**
>
> - Develop a nurse staffing framework based on best available international evidence.
> - Make recommendations for the implementation and monitoring of the framework (including education, training, and guidance).
> - Apply the framework to change nurse staffing at three pilot sites.
> - Evaluate the impact of the framework.
>
> **Nurse Staffing Changes**
>
> - Nurse staffing determined using the measure of nursing hours per patient day.
> - Staffing was increased in understaffed wards.
> - Increased staffing had a stabilising effect and resulted in improved patient, staff, and organisational outcomes.
> - Rostered skill mix reached a level of 80% registered nurses in all wards.
> - 100% of clinical nurse managers' time in most wards was available to supervise and lead others (as opposed to having a direct patient caseload).
>
> **Impact of Applying the Framework**
>
> - Reduced use of agency staff (even in the wards that did not have an uplift).
> - Average patient length of stay shorter (by 2 days or more).
> - Fewer reports of patient care being left undone (from 76% before to 32% after).
> - Improved staff views of the practice environment.
> - Quality of care delivered to patients rated more highly by staff.
>
> Adapted from the Department of Health, Ireland.[67]

2.4 Staffing and Healthcare Improvement

Without adequate staffing and dedicated time, the risk is that improvement work becomes another aspect of service delivery that is neglected or left undone.[68,69] Addressing staff insufficiency depends, of course, on an accurate local assessment of the work to be done and the skills and numbers of staff needed to do it. For example, initiatives such as the Productive Ward, designed to improve quality and in the longer term release time to care, have often been hampered by lack of staff to backfill and enable implementation of change.[70] Staffing fully takes time; improving how care is delivered also takes time; and in healthcare, time means staff. Needleman and Hassmiller argue that goals of assuring the adequacy and performance of hospital nursing, improving quality, and achieving effective cost control need to be thought about collectively and not as competing priorities, noting that:

> ... *simply changing leadership's view of front-line staff or changing hospital culture to embrace a culture of improvement will be insufficient ... improvement must be institutionalized in the day-to-day work of the front-line staff, with adequate time and resources provided and with front-line staff participating in decision making.*[71]

However, even with the right staff in the right place and at the right time, care quality is not guaranteed and improvement is not assured. How staff work together within a team, the extent to which they feel safe to raise concerns and challenge unsafe practices, and the extent to which they are well themselves and able to operate to the best of their abilities also have an impact. Sections 3 and 4 look at these other key building blocks to creating the conditions in which healthcare quality and improvement can be achieved.

3 Psychological Safety, Teamwork, and Speaking Up

Acknowledging and attending to the social and cultural context is vital if improvement interventions are to work.[72] Regardless of the number or mix of staff, *how* staff work together influences the chances of achieving safe, high-quality care and the ability to learn from mistakes. Achieving high-quality care is more dependent than ever on how well people work together; this in turn is affected by organisational factors like leadership and the working environment, not just clinical training.

Psychological safety, teamwork, and speaking up are distinct but interrelated phenomena that affect both the quality of healthcare and the ability to improve it. This section focuses on these three factors as an additional set of workplace conditions that affect healthcare improvement.

- **Psychological safety** is defined as an interpersonal climate in which individuals feel able to take interpersonal risks without fear of negative consequences.[73]
- Psychological safety is considered especially relevant for enabling **speaking up** – a behaviour in which people voice their observations, questions, and concerns, especially to colleagues above them in a hierarchy.[73]

- **Teamwork** describes coordination and collaboration activities through which people accomplish interdependent tasks – as noted in a review of research on teams in healthcare.[74]

3.1 Teams and Psychological Safety

Improvement work necessitates small interpersonal risks – including the risk of looking ignorant (asking a question that might expose your ignorance to others), looking incompetent (when admitting a mistake or a weakness), or appearing negative or critical (when pointing out a flaw in a process worthy of improvement). One way for individuals to minimise risk to their image is simply to remain silent. The problem with this approach is that it precludes learning and innovation.

Similarly, by its very nature, teamwork involves interpersonal risk. Rather than carrying out prescribed tasks with scripted interactions, people working effectively in teams must constantly ask questions, offer ideas, and coordinate actions, with the ever-present risk that actions may not align perfectly and so require continuous attention and adjustment. An important responsibility for healthcare leaders, therefore, is to understand psychological safety, its role in teamwork, and its antecedents.[75–77]

Classic research by Goffman describes how people avoid behaviours that might threaten the image others hold of them,[78] and helps to explain the relationship between psychological safety and teamwork. Social psychologists call this well-documented tendency 'impression management'. Holding back from speaking up with a comment or question that might lead others – especially those in a formal evaluative role – to see us in a negative light is all but second nature for most working adults. The concept of psychological safety was first described in the management literature in the 1960s as a factor in helping people to learn new behaviours and overcome defensive routines.[79] Research on psychological safety has flourished since the turn of the century, in part driven by recognition of its importance in complex, interdependent work.[80] Two meta-analyses compiling empirical evidence of the relationship between psychological safety and team outcomes from more than 80 unique studies have further established the construct as a useful one for organisational research.[75,80] Among the positive outcomes of psychological safety are better communication, knowledge sharing, speaking up, learning behaviour, creativity, innovation, engagement, and performance.

The salience of psychological safety for teamwork and improvement work is well established (see Edmondson and Lei[77] for a review). A lack of psychological safety can be found at the root of many noteworthy organisational errors and failures across industries. A climate of psychological safety, on the other hand, makes it easier for people to voice tentative thoughts. And as team members share ideas, respond respectfully to the views of others, and engage in healthy debate, they establish vital shared expectations about appropriate ways to behave. In particular, a climate of psychological safety can help people override a tendency to default to silence, instead encouraging or allowing them to offer ideas, report errors, and speak up in ways that are vital for healthcare improvement. Improvement starts with clear-eyed identification of quality gaps, including errors and wasteful workarounds (i.e. shortcuts people take at work when they confront a problem that disrupts their ability to carry out a required task). When people feel unable to speak up about such shortcomings, efforts to change work processes for the better are thwarted. A climate of psychological safety may have a particularly important role in efforts to detect errors (e.g. work by Edmondson et al.[81,82]) and in preventing errors before patients are harmed (e.g. Edmondson[81] and Goodman et al.[83]).

Some adverse events occur when a confluence of small process failures combine in unfortunate ways (the Swiss cheese model[84]) that no one anticipates; more often, however, someone experiences a flicker of concern but remains silent for fear of the consequences of speaking up. The real-life episodes in Boxes 4 and 5 illustrate this phenomenon.

Some research has found that groups with higher psychological safety report more errors to head nurses;[81] but crucially, a combination of high psychological safety and nurses' beliefs that patient safety is a high departmental priority is associated with the fewest errors.[89] People can perform the highest quality work and still be willing to talk about the errors that do occur;[81] moreover, this is how high-quality work (error-free, at the sharp end) is achieved in complex settings – by openness and vigilance along the way. By contrast, error rates may be high when psychological safety is low, even when staff believe the department is

---

Box 4 A MICRO-MOMENT OF SILENCE

A nurse on the night shift in a busy urban hospital notices that a dose for a postoperative patient appears not quite right. Fleetingly, he considers calling the doctor at home to check the order but – on recalling her disparaging comments about his abilities last time he had, without a great deal of conscious thought, called her at home – he reconsiders. All but certain that the dose is fine (the patient is on an experimental protocol, after all), he grabs the medication and heads for the patient's bed. This micro-moment of silence depicts what it means to lack psychological safety in the face of uncertainty.

Adapted from Edmondson.[81]

> ### Box 5 Not safe to speak up in a pandemic
>
> During the 2020 COVID-19 pandemic, there were several cases of clinicians speaking up about PPE shortages only to be bullied, rebuked, or fired by their hospitals.[85] Employers had warned that workers should toe the party line and threatened that speaking up will result in positions and careers becoming untenable.[86] Clinicians assumed it was safe to speak up about shortages of lifesaving equipment, only to discover that despite patients' and their own safety being at risk, they were wrong. Mannion and Davies describe a 'well-worn path' where 'concerns about care are raised and ignored, staff are denigrated or bullied and the situation escalates into whistleblowing to outside authorities'.[87] A prolonged neglect of concerns, warning signs, and signals from workers can create deep pockets of organisational silence, 'deafness', and 'blindness'.[88]

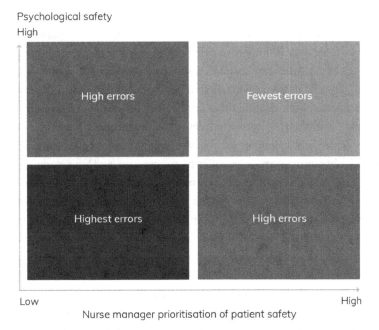

Psychological safety

High

High errors

Fewest errors

Highest errors

High errors

Low High

Nurse manager prioritisation of patient safety

Figure 1 How the relationship between manager prioritisation of patient safety and psychological safety affects organisational errors
Adapted from Leroy et al.[89]

committed to patient safety (see Figure 1).[89] Psychological safety therefore appears to be vital for continuous improvement and to the quality of patient care.

The positive effects of psychological safety on employee engagement have also been established.[90–92] Engagement – the extent to which an employee feels passionate about the job and committed to the organisation – is seen as an index of willingness to put discretionary effort into one's work. Disengagement can lead to safety risks and high staff turnover, which in turn leads to additional recruitment and training costs and a less experienced workforce. Accordingly, interest has grown in improving healthcare working environments as a strategy for employee retention. In one study of clinical staff at a large metropolitan hospital, psychological safety was related both to a commitment to the organisation and patient safety. The authors note that a working environment in which healthcare workers feel safe to speak up about problems is especially important for helping them feel able to provide safe care and be engaged in their work.[93]

3.2 Psychological Safety and Improvement Work

Merely launching improvement projects is insufficient for ensuring progress: supervisors cannot simply command staff to work on such projects without creating a fertile soil of psychological safety to soften the interpersonal risks. A study of more than 100 improvement project teams in neonatal intensive care units in 23 North American hospitals discovered considerable variation in their success.[94] By asking team members to report on what they did to improve unit processes, researchers identified two distinct sets of learning behaviour: 'learn-what' and 'learn-how'. Learn-what describes independent activities, such as reading the medical literature; learn-how comprises team-based learning, such as proactively sharing knowledge, offering suggestions, and brainstorming better approaches. Arguably, both are vital for improvement work. Psychological safety predicted learn-how behaviours (which involve interpersonal risk) but had no statistical relationship with the learn-what activities. This means that while psychological safety is important for behaviours that involve interpersonal risk, it does not adversely affect learning behaviours that you can do alone (e.g. read a book, take an online course).

Relatedly, psychological safety is associated with nurse engagement in improvement work to reduce 'workarounds'.[94,95] A workaround accomplishes the immediate goal but perpetuates the problem that triggered the workaround in the first place. Because workarounds appear to work in the short term, they can delay or prevent process improvement. But the problems that trigger workarounds might more usefully be seen as small signals of a need for change in a system or process. When clinicians do not feel safe enough to speak up and suggest improvements, workarounds are perpetuated. A study of cancer teams found that those with low psychological safety relied more on workarounds, while teams with high psychological safety focused more on diagnosing problems and improving the processes that caused them.[96] Here again, the crucial mechanism that makes it possible to alter and improve work processes is the ease with which people are able to speak up about problems.

3.3 Psychological Safety in the Broader Context

Speaking up at work can, of course, be difficult. People naturally worry that their boss or colleagues will not like what they have to say, so interpersonal risk remains a formidable barrier to effective teamwork and improvement activities. In the several dozen empirical studies of psychological safety, several types of influences on psychological safety have been identified. In rough order of emphasis, they are: leadership behaviour, organisational support, team attributes, relationship networks, and personality factors (see the 2017 review by Newman et al.).[76]

Supportive leadership behaviour is the most prominent factor in promoting psychological safety in a team. In healthcare studies, one of the most frequently identified variables is leadership inclusiveness[97] or the degree to which leaders are perceived as accessible, invite input, and acknowledge their own fallibility. An improvement-oriented management style,[96] behaviour integrity,[89] and shared leadership[98] are also related to psychological safety in teams. Box 6 illustrates the role of leadership in the use of a dry run in an operating theatre. (For further discussion, see the Element on governance and leadership.[100])

Organisational factors that influence psychological safety include perceptions of organisational support,[101] access to mentoring,[102] and diversity practices.[103] Team attributes that influence psychological safety include a climate of continuous

---

BOX 6 FEELING SAFE TO SPEAK UP IN THE OPERATING ROOM

In a study of 16 cardiac surgery departments implementing a new minimally invasive technology, clinicians in some (but not all) of these departments were able to speak up. One practice that helped was a dry run (i.e. with no patient present) to make it easier to practise speaking up despite status differences. In one operating team, a technician reported:

The night before [our first real minimally invasive case] we did everything. . . . We'd had a couple of talks in advance and the night before we walked through the process step by step. . . . We communicated with each other as if it were happening – 'the balloon is going in,' and so on . . . [And, the surgeon] gave us a talk about . . . the kind of communication he wanted in the OR [operating room], what results he expected, and told us to immediately let him know if anything is out of place.

Adapted from Edmonson et al.[99]

> ### Box 7 Not questioning orders
>
> A neonatology nurse wondered why a premature infant was not being given surfactant to promote the high-risk baby's lung development. Stepping forward to remind the doctor about the widely used protocol, she instead caught herself – recalling a public humiliation experienced by another nurse when questioning one of his orders.
>
> Adapted from Edmondson.[108]

improvement (positive) and the existence of subgroups (negative). A growing literature is also investigating the effects of relationship networks on psychological safety. This includes research demonstrating effects on psychological safety of having rewarding co-worker relationships,[104] energising relationships,[105] and prior interaction with team members.[106]

For team leaders and senior clinicians, their own comfort in speaking up is less important for establishing psychological safety than how they respond when *other* members voice concerns, ask for help, or point out an error. Critical events, especially early in a team's life, can have an exaggerated influence on team norms.[107] A single instance of a leader critiquing, talking over, or otherwise dismissing a concern raised by a team member can set a precedent for the whole team and increase the perceived risks of raising such concerns well into the future (see Box 7). It is easy for critical incidents to turn into repeated patterns. And once a norm of not rocking the boat becomes established, it takes serious effort to reverse it.

It is not only leaders who are responsible for creating a healthy climate, however; all employees can help to shape a work environment characterised by candour and commitment to improvement. They do this by taking the very small risks of speaking up with their observations and by asking thoughtful questions that encourage others to do the same.

Overall, a large body of accumulated research suggests that healthcare organisations would do well to emphasise learning and continuous improvement, while providing supportive working conditions and offering training for mid-level leaders (and all people managers) whose behaviours seem to have the most influence on the psychological safety climate in healthcare settings.

4 Staff Health and Well-being at Work

Healthcare staff in many countries around the world, including the UK, work in systems under pressure from workforce shortages, rising patient demand, and increased throughput and work intensity.[109,110] Workplaces may lack adequate resources, effective teamwork, and psychological safety. All these factors can contribute to poor mental and physical well-being, and improvement efforts may be neglected as staff manage day-to-day pressures, firefight in poor working environments, and become stressed and burnt out. This section unpacks the work challenges specific to healthcare; explores the consequences of poor well-being at work, including the link between staff well-being at work and care quality; and identifies interventions to support psychological well-being at work.

4.1 Specific Work Challenges in Healthcare

Healthcare professionals are exposed to a range of emotional and physical challenges in their day-to-day delivery of patient care. Working and learning in the health and care sector is like no other employment environment; staff are confronted daily with extremes of joy, sadness, and despair, and clinical staff may retain traumatic memories.[111] NHS staff are more likely to incur a work-related illness or injury than staff in other sectors,[112] and they have a higher rate of sickness absence compared to the average UK worker (in both the public and private sectors).[113] Stress among healthcare staff is greater than in the general working population and explains more than 25% of absence.[112] Depression, anxiety, and a loss of idealism and empathy are reported by nurses.[114,115] Heavy workloads, bureaucracy, and dealing with challenging patient conditions are all significant contributors to staff well-being,[116] and pressure from budget constraints and staff shortages can take its toll on staff as well as patients.[111,117] The well-being of healthcare practitioners is typically worse than in other professions;[118,119] healthcare staff in the UK have been described as running on empty and the 'shock absorbers in a system lacking [the] resources to meet rising demands'.[117] Many countries in Europe and around the world face similar challenges.[120]

One approach commonly used to understand staff well-being at work is the job demands-resources (JD-R) model.[121] Job demands are physical or emotional stressors, such as time pressures, heavy workloads, difficult working environments, emotional labour, and poor relationships. Job resources (positives) are the physical, social, and organisational factors that help achieve goals and reduce stress – including autonomy, good working relationships, and (peer, supervisor, and team) support. The JD-R model suggests that availability of job and personal resources can help cushion the negative effects of high job demands on employee well-being. Staff with high levels of job discretion and support can be expected to cope more effectively with their job demands, while well-being is likely to be lowest in situations characterised by a combination of high job demands and limited resources.[122] In our own study,[123] which examined links between staff well-being at work and patient experiences of care, we found that high job demands can significantly dampen, if not completely nullify, the positive effect of job and individual resources on well-being; resources are more likely to have a beneficial effect when job demands are less intense.[123]

4.2 The Consequences of Poor Well-being at Work

Without the right support, staff are vulnerable to chronic stress and mental illness,[114] and up to one in three healthcare professionals experiences forms of psychological distress that necessitate clinical intervention.[124] Poor mental health among the NHS workforce is a major healthcare issue, leading to presenteeism, absenteeism, and loss of staff.[111] Emotional exhaustion, burnout, high sickness absence, and high turnover are all common.[125,126] Multiple government and industry reports have highlighted the need to reduce stress and improve mental health among NHS staff.[111,127–129] Neglecting the well-being of healthcare staff also has significant implications for patients; rates of sickness absence among NHS staff are double the national average[113] and are estimated to cost £1.1 billion per annum.[111]

International evidence highlights the consequences of adverse workplace conditions. Research across 12 European countries suggests longer working hours in the nursing profession cause poor well-being and lead to higher rates of burnout and medical risk.[130] Among UK doctors, the effects of work-related stress on sleep, health, and personal relationships have led to early retirement.[131] Several international studies indicate that staff are more likely to intend leaving their profession or to experience absenteeism when they suffer from low well-being or burnout.[132,133] In the UK, the cost to the NHS of the deterioration in staff retention is thought to be as much as £100 million per annum.[111]

Hall et al.'s systematic review synthesised 46 quantitative studies to determine whether well-being and burnout in healthcare professionals is associated with patient safety.[134] Of the 27 studies measuring well-being, 16 found links between poor well-being and poor patient safety. Of the 30 studies measuring burnout, 21 found associations between burnout and patient safety. Poor well-being and moderate-to-high levels of burnout can therefore be linked to poor patient safety outcomes. Patient safety measures often relied on self-reported errors, however. The authors suggest future research could be enhanced by the use of clearer definitions of staff well-being, studies capable of determining causality between concepts, and conducting studies in primary care settings.[134]

More broadly, there is some evidence of associations between staff well-being at work, patient experience, and safety outcomes.[7,123,135] Patient experiences are generally better when staff feel they have a good local team/work group climate, job satisfaction, no emotional exhaustion, a positive organisational climate, and support from co-workers, supervisors, and their organisation. In 2009, the landmark Boorman review found that patient satisfaction in acute trusts was higher where staff health and well-being (measured by injury rates, stress levels, job satisfaction, and turnover intentions) were higher.[112] Conversely, poorer outcomes and patient experiences were likely when staff were unhappy or unhealthy and where there were high rates of staff sickness, stress, and turnover.[112] Staff themselves recognised a link: over 80% of staff who contributed to the Boorman review said their state of health affected patient care. In 2016, a systematic review concluded that 'poor wellbeing and moderate to high levels of burnout are associated, in the majority of studies reviewed, with poor patient safety outcomes such as medical errors' but 'the lack of pro-spective studies reduces the ability to determine causality'.[134]

While the relationship between staff well-being and the delivery of high-quality care makes intuitive sense, it is often simplified as happy staff meaning happy patients (and vice versa).[136-138] Studies now suggest a more complex picture: the well-being and experiences of healthcare staff do influence patient experiences of care for good or ill,[123] but staff happiness and well-being are also shaped by the quality of immediate working relationships[139-141] and staff workplace behaviours towards one another.[142] Our study examining links between staff well-being and patient experiences confirms this, highlighting the importance of the local work climate for staff well-being and high-quality patient care delivery.[123] A strong climate for patient care, particularly at the team level, can help to reinforce some of the positive effects of individual well-being on patient care performance; and crucially, it can also make up for the absence of high levels of individual well-being.

The Boorman review recommended that staff health and well-being should be embedded in the core business of the NHS in order to deliver long-term savings and improved patient care[112] – a recommendation that was adopted in the 2010 NHS white paper. This policy focus seemed overdue then, yet 10 years later the NHS Staff and Learners' Mental Wellbeing Commission noted that levels of staff stress, bullying and harassment, and sickness absence had all increased and appeared intractable.[111]

In 2015 Bodenheimer and Sinsky proposed expanding the Institute for Healthcare Improvement's Triple Aim framework, whose three aims – enhan-cing patient experience, improving population health, and reducing costs – are widely accepted as a compass for optimising health system performance. Bodenheimer and Sinsky's proposal was for a quadruple aim, adding the goal of improving the work life of healthcare providers, including clinicians and staff.[143] We endorse this, but we suggest it is important to go beyond the system level that the authors address: improving the work life and psychological well-being of healthcare staff is important in its own right and imperative for good employers and individual staff members and their teams.

4.3 Interventions to Support Psychological Well-being at Work

The well-being of healthcare staff is now firmly on the international agenda, but evidence is limited for which well-being interventions are most appropriate for different staff groups working in different environments. A key debate continues to centre on whether interventions should be individually or organisationally focused – or perhaps both. A 2019 review commissioned by the Department of Health concluded that interventions need to operate at an organisational level and have the commitment and engagement of senior staff in order to improve working conditions.[114] In practice and research, however, interventions are frequently geared towards improving individual coping mechanisms, such as mindfulness training, resilience building, and mentoring.[144,145]

4.3.1 Individual Interventions

In terms of an individual focus, there is some evidence to suggest that mindfulness has good outcomes. A 2017 systematic review analysed the evidence on mindfulness-based interventions and their effectiveness in reducing stress among healthcare professionals. It concluded that such interventions may reduce stress, but the evidence is limited because of small sample sizes and lack of theoretical framing; longer-term follow-ups are required.[146] Lomas et al.'s 2018 review found that mindfulness interventions are associated with positive outcomes, and this appears to be a consistent finding across different healthcare professions, including mental health staff. But mindfulness is constructed in a number of ways across the studies, and only 26 of the 66 studies involved a control group, which make conclusions about well-being improvement difficult to compare.[147]

Some evidence supports clinical supervision in the helping professions,[148] including a controlled trial with mental health nurses in Australia[149] and restorative supervision with public health nurses in the UK.[150] The latter seeks to overcome some of the challenges that have become inherent in clinical supervision – the risk that it becomes a managerial approach to oversight and professional surveillance rather than an educational therapeutic space for staff to process and make sense of challenging clinical encounters. Drawing on the evidence to develop interventions to support staff psychologically during the COVID-19 pandemic, we have identified a range of evidence-informed interventions for individuals, teams, managers, and leaders, including the importance of peer support, buddying, and places to reflect on and make sense of practice with colleagues.[151] Most are also relevant for supporting healthcare staff during non-pandemic times.

There is less good evidence regarding the resilience-based training programmes that have become commonplace in healthcare.[152,153] Traynor delivers a blistering critique of resilience training and resilience as a concept used in nursing to explore the factors that enable nurses to overcome adversity.[154] He argues that warnings from leaders in the field of resilience research have not been heeded; they suggest resilience is not simply an individual's inner quality but is linked to systems/contexts and the individual's response to these.[154] An overemphasis on nurses being resilient in the face of understaffing and often intense emotional work is consistently challenged by nurses and nurse academics, who see the framing and targeting of resilience as an individual trait as letting organisations 'off the hook'.[154] Too often, however, an individualistic focus on resilience has been the primary strategy of healthcare organisations to date.

4.3.2 Organisation or System-Wide Interventions

Carrieri et al.'s[155] analysis of 179 studies of doctors (45% from the USA) found that interventions that emphasise relationships and belonging, such as those creating a people-focused working culture, were more likely to promote well-being, concluding that multidimensional and multilevel interventions to tackle doctors' and students' mental ill health are most likely to be successful.[155] Generally, however, the focus on organisation-wide or system-wide interventions – addressing, for example, job redesign and task restructuring – has been lacking (notwithstanding the Magnet hospitals discussed in Section 2.3.1).[156] One systematic review of interventions that included all healthcare staff within a healthcare setting (e.g. the whole hospital or a whole unit/ward) in collective activities to improve physical or mental health or promote healthy behaviours identified just 11 studies that used a whole-system approach.[118] Yet these very structural aspects of work are precisely those identified by proponents of the quadruple aim[143,157] and those who have studied poor mental health among healthcare professionals.[118]

One organisation-wide intervention that shows promise is Schwartz Rounds (often referred to as simply Rounds), where issues of emotional, social, and ethical complexity are examined and questions and issues about healthcare quality can be explored. Rounds are open to all staff in a healthcare organisation and provide a (usually monthly) forum to discuss the emotional impact of work in a safe and confidential environment.[158,159] Rounds are widely used in the USA and have grown in popularity in healthcare organisations in the UK, Ireland, and Australia. Rounds last 1 hour and commence with three-to-four staff stories presenting an experience that is collectively shared (e.g. a patient case), or a set of individual experiences based around a theme (e.g. a patient I'll never forget). Staff tell stories that reflect complex issues, which can provide learning for colleagues and enable ripple effects and changes in practice to occur (see Box 8 for an example).[158]

Taylor et al. synthesised evidence for Rounds and compared their effectiveness to other reflective interventions, such as action learning sets, after action reviews, and Balint groups.[124] Prior to Maben et al.'s 2018 evaluation undertaken in the UK,[158] however, evidence for their effectiveness was limited. Though studies had determined that Rounds were highly valued by attendees, most used non-validated questionnaires and had weak designs with no control group.[124] Maben et al. used a realist evaluation approach with nine case studies and a survey with control group. The survey found that poor psychological well-being (measured by the clinically validated GHQ-12) reduced significantly more in Rounds attenders (a 13% decrease compared with 3% in non-attenders). Among regular Rounds attenders, poor psychological well-being

---

BOX 8 SCHWARTZ ROUNDS: SHARING AND HEARING OTHER STAFF EXPERIENCES
CHANGES BEHAVIOUR

A doctor reported hearing colleagues present a story about a vulnerable patient being discharged too soon. He said:

I suppose what's had the biggest impact on the way I provide compassionate care and what's changed my behaviour the most is the Round where we had the vulnerable adults team presenting. They presented a story in great detail about a patient, who was medically fit for discharge and therefore perceived by the trust as a 'bed-blocker', but actually they were very vulnerable and they couldn't be safely discharged and what had happened when they'd been discharged inappropriately in the past. For me that's the situation in which I am most commonly at risk of not providing compassionate care like last night when the hospital has no beds – it was remembering those stories about the risks of sending home vulnerable adults that has made me stop and think. That is the Round that's changed my behaviour to the greatest extent.

Adapted from Maben et al.[158]

dropped from 25% to 12%, compared with a non-significant reduction (37% to 34%) in those who chose not to attend Rounds (the control group). Other reported outcomes include a greater understanding of context and therefore insights into the behaviour of colleagues, patients, and caregivers, which resulted in increased tolerance, empathy, and compassion for colleagues and patients. Better support for staff, reduced isolation, improved teamwork and communication, and reported changes in practice were also noted.[158]

Rounds could provide a psychologically safe space in which issues of quality, safety, and healthcare improvement could be identified and foregrounded, and organisational behaviour change could be reported (see Box 9 for an example). Rounds are not for everyone, however; some staff struggled to attend, in particular ward-based nurses and community staff.[158]

As we have shown, however, the evidence on intervention effectiveness in terms of improving staff well-being is limited, particularly for interventions involving whole-system approaches (i.e. those that consider both individual and organisational factors) as recommended in the Boorman review.[112] Further, the evidence is often compiled from global sources (e.g. Hall et al.[134] and Burton et al.[146]), thereby neglecting the different contexts of different health systems. Though somewhat constrained, the evidence base that exists on whole-system interventional approaches identifies some that appear to be effective.[114,118,124] We have identified one such example, Schwartz Rounds, and provided examples of how in small, but crucially important, ways staff can be engaged, behaviours can be changed, and outcomes identified that improve care quality. In practice, many interventions that target NHS staff place the burden for good mental health on individuals and exhort them to improve their resilience.[151] This neglects the wider structural and organisational constraints and contexts that may have a detrimental effect on staff well-being.[118] We are not suggesting this is an either/or; individual interventions and structural interventions are both important, but not the former without the latter. Overall, we suggest that changing the work environment to promote positive staff well-being at work

---

Box 9 A NEW SUPPORT GROUP SET UP FOR STAFF AS A RESULT OF A SCHWARTZ ROUND

On the back of the Schwartz Round, a colleague emailed the head of nursing. The start of the email read: 'I attended the Schwartz Round, the panel was all nurses and I heard the stories about nurses feeling unsupported and isolated.' As a result, the head of nursing took it up to the board, who agreed to reintroduce clinical supervision for nurses.

Adapted from Maben et al.[158]

is likely to better enable quality, safety, and improvement work; the benefits are not just an absence of negatives (sickness absence, low morale, high turnover) but an enriched and motivated staff more able to fully engage in their work and improve quality.

5 Conclusions

This Element has focused on the workforce and people dimensions of health-care improvement, seeking to identify the conditions required to enable staff to engage in their work and improve quality. We have considered how workplace conditions influence the work of improvement and the creation of an optimal culture for improvement where, every day and at every level, the work context must support the question, 'how could we do this better?' Fostering conditions that allow staff to flourish and contribute – not just to delivering current services but to continuously improving them – is vital, especially given that in many countries recruiting, supporting, and retaining the healthcare workforce is a major challenge. The NHS People Plan makes this clear: it seeks to make the NHS an employer of excellence and an excellent place to work, improving culture so that staff feel they have fulfilment, voice, and belonging.[160] All three of the conditions for healthcare improvement that we identify – staffing adequacy, psychological safety, and staff well-being – depend on leadership, management support, and role modelling. We have drawn on a wide range of evidence to suggest that without attention to the needs of the workforce and to workplace conditions, many improvement interventions or approaches may fail – either because staff are not engaged and actively involved, or because the causes and consequences of poor workplace conditions for staff and for improvement are not given sufficient attention.

5.1 Quality Is the Mainstay of Healthcare Professionals' Work

Healthcare staff often want more than the opportunity (and resources) to deliver excellent care. They want to use their skills, knowledge, and expertise to improve the quality of care provided. We agree with Needleman and Hassmiller that improving healthcare 'must be institutionalized in the day-to-day work of the front-line staff, with adequate time and resources provided and with front-line staff participating in decision making'.[71] This positioning of quality as the mainstay of the work of healthcare professionals thus needs to be reflected in the systems and contexts that healthcare organisations themselves provide and create: the vision for quality and constant improvement should be clear, the resources and training required should be available, and the context should be enabling. Part of enablement involves providing staff and patients with the resources, opportunities, and skills they need to contribute. Recognition of this often manifests in drives from senior leadership or management to build improvement capability; but frontline staff and service users must also feel able to make use of these skills and take ownership of improvement work.[161]

Staff are more likely to come forward with system improvements when there is a culture that supports voicing concerns and speaking up,[87,162] in particular where a culture of psychological safety is encouraged.[163] When teams feel psychologically safe, they share information of significance. They make decisions collectively and perform better together, thereby improving patient safety.[73,164] In a healthcare setting, psychological safety enables learning, experimentation, and the production of new practices[73] – factors that have been shown to reduce patient mortality rates.[94,165] Linked to this, it is important to recognise how problems of quality and safety are identified, defined, and selected for attention, by whom, through which power structures, and with what consequences – and how the exclusion of some healthcare workers from these processes may be hampering improvements in care for patients.[166]

The question of how to create conditions that will enable healthcare improvement – rather than it being seen as an add-on or becoming one more activity that is left undone due to time pressures – connects with themes about embedding strategies for quality in the culture of an organisation (as described in the Element on making culture change happen[167]). Organisations also need to grasp the relationships between workplace conditions and improvement and that these relationships potentially work in both directions: good workplace conditions enable improvement, but improvement work (and enabling staff to engage in it) may create system efficiencies that then improve workplace conditions, thereby enabling better staff well-being, greater psychological safety, and optimum staffing, which results in a reduction of the workload burden on staff.

We conclude by drawing together the main themes and insights from all sections (see Table 1) to inform organisations' thinking about how best to create the necessary conditions to capitalise on their most valuable asset in pursuit of improvement in healthcare: their people.

5.2 A Future Research Agenda

Despite the significance of the workforce and people dimensions of quality and safety and their centrality as structural conditions, the healthcare improvement literature has to date paid insufficient attention to the three conditions we have outlined in this Element – staffing adequacy, psychological safety, and staff well-being. In Box 10, we identify what might be done to address the gaps in the literature.

Table 1 Workplace conditions and healthcare improvement

Workplace Condition	Key Issues	Implications for Quality and Improvement	Assessment: How Do You Know If You've Got It Right?
Staffing *A relationship between the number and skills of staff delivering care and the attainment of care quality, or the ability to improve it, is irrefutable*	• Most existing evidence is on nurse staffing; there is little evidence for other staff groups. • Research supports the plausibility of a causal link between registered nurse staffing, care quality, and patient outcomes. • Missed registered nurse care partially mediates the relationship between registered nurse staffing and avoidable patient mortality. • Little specificity exists about how many registered nurses is enough.	Low levels of registered nurses are associated with: • more adverse patient events • increased length of stay • higher rates of death and falls • more missed care • nurse burnout and poor well-being • lower staff engagement.	• Use nursing workload measurement tools, e.g. NICE-endorsed Safer Nursing Care Tool.[36] • Finding suitable, meaningful, and feasible nursing care quality measures is a recognised challenge. • Seek to investigate staffing and staff workload issues in relation to care quality and outcomes or process measures such as care left undone.

Psychological Safety
Psychological safety, teamwork, and speaking up are inter-related and critical for healthcare improvement

- Education of nursing staff and skill mix makes a difference.
- The international shortage of registered nurses is ongoing.
- Staffing is about more than numbers; practice environments are also critically important.
- A climate where individuals are able to take interpersonal risks without fear of negative consequences is highly important.
- Numerous studies highlight the need for psychological safety in healthcare.
- Healthcare leaders must understand psychological safety and its role in teamwork.

- Psychological safety promotes efforts to detect errors so as to prevent harm; it helps people catch and correct errors that may happen before patients are harmed.
- Quality of care is more dependent than ever on how well people work together.
- Improvement work necessitates small interpersonal risks (e.g. looking ignorant or

- Consider psychological safety measurement survey measures – e.g. 7-point scale.[94]
- Use confidential hypothetical scenarios with questions to gather data.
- Link psychological safety measurement with safety outcomes.
- Reflect on and evaluate culture: set the stage for psychological safety; respond

Table 1 (cont.)

Workplace Condition	Key Issues	Implications for Quality and Improvement	Assessment: How Do You Know If You've Got It Right?
	• Staff in psychologically unsafe workplaces may not speak up, for example, about issues of quality and safety.	incompetent, seeming negative or critical).	productively to make it happen;[108] make it safe to fail; motivate a staff learning mindset with situational humility and proactive inquiry (powerful questions); express appreciation; destigmatise failure; create cultures to elicit ideas and concerns.
Well-being at Work *It is the experience of healthcare staff that shapes patient experiences of care for good or ill, not the other way around*[123]	• Healthcare staff experience extremes of joy, sadness, and despair, resulting in high financial/personal costs relating to well-being at work. • Well-being of healthcare staff is typically worse than in other professions (higher work-related illness or injury,	• Without good staff engagement and well-being, healthcare improvement issues are neglected as staff seek to manage the day-to-day pressures, leaving them firefighting in poor working environments and feeling stressed and burnt out.	• Monitor patient experience (e.g. complaints and real-time feedback) and staff well-being (e.g. high sickness absence, reports of bullying, annual staff surveys) to: ◦ target resources to areas that are known to be problematic

higher rate of sickness absence and stress).

- Interventions targeting individual staff neglect the wider structural and organisational constraints/contexts.

Overall Issues

Improvement must be institutionalised in the day-to-day work of frontline staff, with adequate time and resources provided and with frontline staff participating in decision-making[71]

- Evidence to suggest staff well-being at work is associated with patient experience and safety outcomes.

- Some professional groups engage with healthcare improvement more than others.
- Nurses are not necessarily well prepared to undertake improvement work, nor given responsibility to do so.
- Healthcare improvement can be an activity undertaken by experts and early adopters, in isolation from their peers.

  o disseminate learning in good practice from teams and groups that are doing well
  o implement team/organisational and individual interventions in tandem (not just individual interventions alone).

- Improvement work needs to provide opportunity and skills to contribute.
- Recognition of this need often manifests in drives from senior leadership or management to build healthcare improvement capability in healthcare organisations, but it also requires that frontline staff and service users feel able to make use of these

- Examine how quality and safety problems are identified/defined/selected for attention by whom, through which power structures, and with what consequences.
- Create the conditions to avoid improvement work being seen as an add-on; embed strategies for quality in the culture of an organisation and provide resources.

Table 1 (cont.)

Workplace Condition	Key Issues	Implications for Quality and Improvement	Assessment: How Do You Know If You've Got It Right?
	• Staff need to *see* quality, and their part in *improving* it, as part of their individual and team's roles. • Healthcare professionals need to have skills and competences to engage in improvement and beyond 'getting the job done'.	skills and take ownership of such work. • Quality and healthcare improvement training for healthcare professionals tends to be uni-disciplinary, whereas the importance of teams and of understanding and supporting each other at work is crucial.	• Improving quality and safety is everyone's business and the mainstay of healthcare professionals' work; it needs the vision for quality and constant improvement to be clear, training to be enhanced, the resources to be present, and the context to be enabling.

Box 10 FUTURE RESEARCH RECOMMENDATIONS

Research on the Interaction between the Three Preconditions and Improvement

Develop and fund longitudinal, multidisciplinary research programmes that examine the impact of staffing adequacy, psychological safety, and staff well-being on healthcare improvement – individually and collectively. Specifically, develop and fund studies that:

- investigate the role of emotion work in the development and implementation of improvement work
- focus on increasing workforce capacity for improving care by clarifying the staff time and skills required
- explore the value of a richer skill mix for optimal improvement work
- explore the role of psychological safety (the impact of speak-up cultures and bullying and incivility, for example) in enabling improvement
- tease out how the three preconditions together impact on the successful implementation of improvement interventions
- evaluate the impact of healthcare improvement on staff well-being at work (e.g. on stress, burnout, engagement, morale, and motivation) and the potential workforce benefits (increased job satisfaction and retention).

Research to Address Each of the Three Preconditions

Specifically, staffing research should include:

- more longitudinal staffing research, examining a range of different professional groups
- further staffing research studies outside acute general hospital wards
- better economic analyses in relation to staffing and outcomes (to identify the cost benefits of better staffing)
- system changes in the measurement of outcomes associated with care (better metrics)
- more workforce research that examines the full multidisciplinary team including the medical workforce.

Specifically, psychological safety research should include:

- research on the effects of interventions designed to increase psychological safety

- more research on differences in psychological safety across role groups and organisational levels in healthcare organisations
- studies of changes in psychological safety as a result of changes in workload, staffing levels, burnout, or crisis.

Specifically, well-being research should include:

- clearer definitions of healthcare staff well-being
- more and better evaluation of interventions that support staff well-being
- research outside of acute care – for example, in primary care settings
- studies capable of determining causality between concepts.

6 Further Reading

Staffing for Quality

- Griffiths et al.[15] – a systematic review of the evidence on staffing levels and skill mix, which was commissioned by NICE to help inform the development of safe-staffing guidelines for adult inpatient care. Only studies that measured staffing at a unit level and considered both registered nurse and support worker staffing were included.
- Ball[168] – a special collection editorial weaving together different perspectives on the question of whether we have enough nurses, why the question matters, and disincentives to addressing it.
- Maben et al.[64] – a review commissioned by the Chief Nursing Officer for England, recognising that measurement lies at the heart of efforts to improve care quality and meaningful metrics are key to this.
- National Institute for Health Research (NIHR)[169] – a review summarising evidence from 22 research studies (funded by the NIHR) on planning nurse staffing, skill mix, and the organisation of nursing on hospital wards, with a concise overview of lessons learnt.
- Department of Health, Ireland[67] – a rare example of a framework for safe nurse staffing that includes reference to the cost and investment needed to enable an overall increase in staffing, and also sets out the expected return/benefits on this investment.

Psychological Safety

- Edmondson[108] – a definitive guide to understanding psychological safety, why it matters in the modern workplace, and how to create more of it.

Includes a review of the research literature, more than 20 case studies to bring the ideas to life, and practical tips.

- Edmondson[170] – a book focusing on 'teaming' as a set of coordinating and collaborating behaviours, rather than examining teams as structures. It explains that most teams in today's workplace, especially in healthcare, lack stable, well-bounded membership and provides tips for how to foster effective teaming.
- Burns et al. (editors)[171] – the seventh edition of Shortell and Kaluzny's textbook includes more than a dozen literature reviews and case studies on critical topics to help today's healthcare managers understand and support success in the modern healthcare delivery ecosystem.

Staff Health and Well-being

- Boorman[112] – a comprehensive and seminal review of the well-being of healthcare staff, providing a succinct review of the evidence and a strategy for improving NHS staff well-being at work.
- Brand et al.[118] – a systematic review of the health and well-being of health-care workers, advocating for a whole-system (as opposed to an individual) approach to intervention development.
- Health Education England[111] – an accessible report from a commission that was set up to examine staff and learner well-being in the NHS. It includes an evidence review and testimonies from staff and families of NHS staff bereaved by suicide.
- Taylor et al.[124] – a systematic review of the evidence supporting Schwartz Rounds and a scoping review comparing Rounds to other well-being interventions that use reflection on practice as a process for support.

Contributors

All authors of this Element were involved in the conceptualisation, curation of included materials, and writing of the original draft, as well as reviewing and editing. Jill Maben drafted the introduction, discussion, and wrote the section on staff well-being, and coordinated the preparation of the manuscript. Jane Ball wrote the section on staffing, and Amy C. Edmondson wrote the section on psychological safety. Jane Ball and Amy C. Edmondson contributed to the review and revisions of the original drafts, providing critical comments and edits. All authors have approved the final version.

Conflicts of Interest

Jill Maben was a member of an advisory group in 2006–09, advising on the development of the Point of Care project at The King's Fund, and a member of the Point of Care Foundation Board in 2013–14; she stepped down as board member at the start of the Schwartz Rounds evaluation. Jill Maben was also a member of the Engagement and Involvement Advisory Board of THIS Institute (The Healthcare Improvement Studies Institute) during 2019–22. Jane Ball and Amy C. Edmondson have no conflict of interests to declare.

Acknowledgements

We thank Dr Ruth Abrams for some early insights in the staff well-being evidence base, Sara Nicholson for retrieving papers and providing administrative support for Amy C. Edmondson, Susan Salter for editing support and text refinement, and the peer reviewers for their insightful comments and recommendations to improve the Element. A list of peer reviewers is published at www.cambridge.org/IQ-peer-reviewers.

Funding

This Element was funded by THIS Institute (www.thisinstitute.cam.ac.uk). THIS Institute is strengthening the evidence base for improving the quality and safety of healthcare. THIS Institute is supported by a grant to the University of Cambridge from the Health Foundation – an independent charity committed to bringing about better health and healthcare for people in the UK.

About the Authors

Jill Maben is Professor of Health Services Research and Nursing at the University of Surrey. Jill is a nurse and social scientist and her research focuses on the psychological well-being of staff at work to support them to care well for patients.

Jane Ball is Professor of Nursing Workforce Policy at the University of Southampton. Jane has been researching nurse staffing and workforce policy since 1990. A major interest is nurse staffing levels and the interface between research evidence and policy development.

Amy C. Edmondson, the Novartis Professor of Leadership and Management at Harvard Business School, studies psychological safety and teaming in healthcare delivery and other organisations.

Creative Commons License

The online version of this work is published under a Creative Commons licence called CC-BY-NC-ND 4.0 (https://creativecommons.org/licenses/by-nc-nd/4.0). It means that you're free to reuse this work. In fact, we encourage it. We just ask that you acknowledge THIS Institute as the creator, you don't distribute a modified version without our permission, and you don't sell it or use it for any activity that generates revenue without our permission. Ultimately, we want our work to have impact. So if you've got a use in mind but you're not sure it's allowed, just ask us at enquiries@thisinstitute.cam.ac.uk.

The printed version is subject to statutory exceptions and to the provisions of relevant licensing agreements, so you will need written permission from Cambridge University Press to reproduce any part of it.

All versions of this work may contain content reproduced under licence from third parties. You must obtain permission to reproduce this content from these third parties directly.

References

1. Donabedian A. The quality of care: how can it be assessed? *JAMA* 1988; 260: 1743–8. https://doi.org/10.1001/jama.1988.03410120089033.

2. Kane RL, Shamliyan TA, Mueller C, Duval S, Wilt TJ. The association of registered nurse staffing levels and patient outcomes: systematic review and meta-analysis. *Med Care* 2007; 45: 1195–204. https://doi.org/10.1097/MLR.0b013e3181468ca3.

3. Heinen MM, van Achterberg T, Schwendimann R, et al. Nurses' intention to leave their profession: a cross sectional observational study in 10 European countries. *Int J Nurs Stud* 2013; 50: 174–84. https://doi.org/10.1016/j.ijnurstu.2012.09.019.

4. Duffield C, Buchan J, North N. Nurse turnover: a literature review – an update. *Int J Nurs Stud* 2012; 49: 887–905. https://doi.org/10.1016/j.ijnurstu.2011.10.001.

5. Griffiths P, Dall'Ora C, Ball J. Nurse staffing levels, quality and outcomes of care in NHS hospital wards: what does the evidence say? *Health Work: Evidence Briefs* 2017; 1. http://eprints.soton.ac.uk/id/eprint/412518 (accessed 14 October 2021).

6. Dall'Ora C, Ball J, Reinius M, Griffiths P. Burnout in nursing: a theoretical review. *Hum Resour Health* 2020; 18: 1–17. https://doi.org/10.1186/s12960-020-00469-9.

7. Maben J, Adams M, Peccei R, Murrells T, Robert G. 'Poppets and parcels': the links between staff experience of work and acutely ill older peoples' experience of hospital care. *Int J Older People Nurs* 2012; 7: 83–94. https://doi.org/10.1111/j.1748-3743.2012.00326.x.

8. Rosenstein AH, O'Daniel M. Disruptive behavior and clinical outcomes: perceptions of nurses and physicians. *Am J Nurs* 2005; 105: 54–64. http://doi.org/10.1097/00000446-200501000-00025.

9. Bond C, Raehl CL, Pitterle ME, Franke T. Health care professional staffing, hospital characteristics, and hospital mortality rates. *Pharmacotherapy* 1999; 19: 130–8. https://doi.org/10.1592/phco.19.3.130.30915.

10. Jarman B, Gault S, Alves B, et al. Explaining differences in English hospital death rates using routinely collected data. *BMJ* 1999; 318: 1515–20. https://doi.org/10.1136/bmj.318.7197.1515.

11. West E, Barron DN, Harrison D, et al. Nurse staffing, medical staffing and mortality in intensive care: an observational study. *Int J Nurs Stud* 2014; 51: 781–94. https://doi.org/10.1016/j.ijnurstu.2014.02.007.

12. Albanese MP, Evans DA, Schantz CA, et al. Engaging clinical nurses in quality and performance improvement activities. *Nurs Adm Q* 2010; 34: 226–45. https://doi.org/10.1097/NAQ.0b013e3181e702ca.

13. Draper DA, Felland LE, Liebhaber A, Melichar L. The role of nurses in hospital quality improvement. *Res Brief* 2008; 3: 1–8. www.hschange.org/CONTENT/972/972.pdf (accessed 14 October 2021).

14. Shekelle PG. Nurse-patient ratios as a patient safety strategy: a systematic review. *Ann Intern Med* 2013; 158: 404–9. http://doi.org/10.7326/0003-4819-158-5-201303051-00007.

15. Griffiths P, Ball J, Drennan J, et al. Nurse staffing and patient outcomes: strengths and limitations of the evidence to inform policy and practice. A review and discussion paper based on evidence reviewed for the National Institute for Health and Care Excellence Safe Staffing guideline development. *Int J Nurs Stud* 2016; 63: 213–25. http://doi.org/10.1016/j.ijnurstu.2016.03.012.

16. Aiken LH, Sloane D, Griffiths P, et al. Nursing skill mix in European hospitals: cross-sectional study of the association with mortality, patient ratings, and quality of care. *BMJ Qual Saf* 2017; 26: 559–68. https://doi.org/10.1136/bmjqs-2016-005567.

17. Ausserhofer D, Zander B, Busse R, et al. Prevalence, patterns and predictors of nursing care left undone in European hospitals: results from the multicountry cross-sectional RN4CAST study. *BMJ Qual Saf* 2014; 23: 126–35. https://doi.org/10.1136/bmjqs-2013-002318.

18. Bowers L, Crowder M. Nursing staff numbers and their relationship to conflict and containment rates on psychiatric wards – a cross sectional time series Poisson regression study. *Int J Nurs Stud* 2012; 49: 15–20. http://doi.org/10.1016/j.ijnurstu.2011.07.005.

19. Cook RM, Jones S, Williams GC, et al. An observational study on the rate of reporting of adverse event on healthcare staff in a mental health setting: an application of Poisson expectation maximisation analysis on nurse staffing data. *Health Informatics J* 2019; 26: 1333–46. https://doi.org/10.1177/1460458219874637.

20. Spilsbury K, Hewitt C, Stirk L, Bowman C. The relationship between nurse staffing and quality of care in nursing homes: a systematic review. *Int J Nurs Stud* 2011; 48: 732–50. https://doi.org/10.1016/j.ijnurstu.2011.02.014.

21. Murrells T, Ball J, Maben J, Ashworth M, Griffiths P. Nursing consultations and control of diabetes in general practice: a retrospective observational study. *Br J Gen Pract* 2015; 65: e642–8. https://doi.org/10.3399/bjgp15X686881.

22. Griffiths P, Murrells T, Dawoud D, Jones S. Hospital admissions for asthma, diabetes and COPD: is there an association with practice nurse staffing? A cross sectional study using routinely collected data. *BMC Health Serv Res* 2010; 10: 276. https://doi.org/10.1186/1472-6963-10-276.

23. Griffiths P, Ball J, Drennan J, et al. *The Association between Patient Safety Outcomes and Nurse / Healthcare Assistant Skill Mix and Staffing Levels & Factors That May Influence Staffing Requirements.* National Nursing Research Unit, University of Southampton; 2014. www.nice.org.uk/guidance/sg1/documents/safe-staffing-for-nursing-in-adult-inpatient-wards-in-acute-hospitals-evidence-review-12 (accessed 13 April 2022).

24. Ball JE, Griffiths P. Consensus Development Project (CDP): an overview of staffing for safe and effective nursing care. *Nursing Open* 2022; 9: 872–9. https://doi.org/10.1002/nop2.989.

25. Aiken LH, Sloane DM, Bruyneel L, et al. Nurse staffing and education and hospital mortality in nine European countries: a retrospective observational study. *Lancet* 2014; 383: 1824–30. https://doi.org/10.1016/S0140-6736(13)62631-8.

26. Shang J, Needleman J, Liu J, Larson E, Stone PW. Nurse staffing and healthcare-associated infection, unit-level analysis. *J Nurs Adm* 2019; 49: 260–5. https://doi.org/10.1097/NNA.0000000000000748.

27. Griffiths P, Maruotti A, Saucedo AR, et al. Nurse staffing, nursing assistants and hospital mortality: retrospective longitudinal cohort study. *BMJ Qual Saf* 2019; 28: 609–17. https://doi.org/10.1136/bmjqs-2018-008043.

28. Needleman J, Buerhaus P, Pankratz VS, et al. Nurse staffing and inpatient hospital mortality. *N Engl J Med* 2011; 364: 1037–45. https://doi.org/10.1056/NEJMsa1001025.

29. Ball JE, Murrells T, Rafferty AM, Morrow E, Griffiths P. 'Care left undone' during nursing shifts: associations with workload and perceived quality of care. *BMJ Qual Saf* 2014; 23: 116–25. https://doi.org/10.1136/bmjqs-2012-001767.

30. Sermeus W, Aiken LH, Van den Heede K, et al. Nurse forecasting in Europe (RN4CAST): rationale, design and methodology. *BMC Nurs* 2011; 10: 6. https://doi.org/10.1186/1472-6955-10-6.

31. Ball JE, Bruyneel L, Aiken LH, et al. Post-operative mortality, missed care and nurse staffing in nine countries: a cross-sectional study. *Int J Nurs Stud* 2018; 78: 10–15. https://doi.org/10.1016/j.ijnurstu.2017.08.004.

32. Griffiths P, Ball J, Bloor K, et al. Nurse staffing levels, missed vital signs and mortality in hospitals: retrospective longitudinal observational study. *Health Serv Deliv Res* 2018; 6: 38. https://doi.org/10.3310/hsdr06380.

33. University of Southampton. Research Project. Nurse staffing levels, missed vital signs observations and mortality in hospital wards: modelling the

consequences and costs of variations in nurse staffing and skill mix – Dormant. www.southampton.ac.uk/healthsciences/research/projects/ nurse-staffing-levels-missed-vital-signs.page (accessed 14 October 2021).

34. Griffiths P, Recio-Saucedo A, Dall'Ora C, et al. The association between nurse staffing and omissions in nursing care: a systematic review. *J Adv Nurs* 2018; 74: 1474–87. https://doi.org/10.1111/jan.13564.

35. Recio-Saucedo A, Dall'Ora C, Maruotti A, et al. What impact does nursing care left undone have on patient outcomes? Review of the literature. *J Clin Nurs* 2018; 27: 2248–59. https://doi.org/10.1111/jocn.14058.

36. National Institute for Health and Care Excellence. *Safe Staffing for Nursing in Adult Inpatient Wards in Acute Hospitals: Safe Staffing Guideline (SG1)*. London: NICE; 2014. www.nice.org.uk/guidance/sg1 (accessed 14 October 2021).

37. Department of Health and Social Care. *Guidance: The NHS Constitution for England*. London: DHSC; updated 1 January 2021. www.gov.uk/government/ publications/the-nhs-constitution-for-england/the-nhs-constitution-for-england (accessed 14 October 2021).

38. Nursing and Midwifery Council. *The Code: Professional Standards of Practice and Behaviour for Nurses, Midwives and Nursing Associates*. London: NMC; 2018. www.nmc.org.uk/standards/code (accessed 14 October 2021).

39. Royal College of Nursing. *Mandatory Nurse Staffing Levels (Policy Briefing 03/12)*. London: RCN; 2012. www.rcn.org.uk/about-us/our-influencing-work/policy-briefings/pol-0312 (accessed 14 October 2021).

40. Aiken LH, Sloane DM, Cimiotti JP, et al. Implications of the California nurse staffing mandate for other states. *Health Serv Res* 2010; 45: 904–21. https://doi.org/10.1111/j.1475-6773.2010.01114.x.

41. Gerdtz M, Nelson S. 5–20: a model of minimum nurse-to-patient ratios in Victoria, Australia. *J Nurs Manag* 2007; 15: 64–71. https://doi.org/ 10.1111/j.1365-2934.2006.00657.x.

42. Buchan J. A certain ratio? The policy implications of minimum staffing ratios in nursing. *J Health Serv Res Policy* 2005; 10: 239–44. https://doi .org/10.1258/135581905774414204.

43. Department of Health, Social Services and Public Safety, Northern Ireland. *Delivering Care: Nurse Staffing in Northern Ireland*. Belfast: DHSSPSNI; 2014. www.health-ni.gov.uk/publications/delivering-care-nurse-staffing-levels-northern-ireland (accessed 14 October 2021).

44. Care Quality Commission. *Health and Social Care Act 2008 (Regulated Activities) Regulations 2014: Regulation 18: Staffing*. www.cqc.org.uk/ guidance-providers/regulations-enforcement/regulation-18-staffing (accessed 14 October 2021).

45. Francis R. *Report of the Mid Staffordshire NHS Foundation Trust Public Inquiry: Executive Summary.* London: The Stationery Office; 2013. www .gov.uk/government/publications/report-of-the-mid-staffordshire-nhs-foun dation-trust-public-inquiry (accessed 14 October 2021).

46. Ball J. Staffing ratios of 1:8 indicate "danger", not a safe minimum. *Nurs Times*; 28 May 2014. www.nursingtimes.net/archive/jane-ball-staffing-ratios-of-18-indicate-danger-not-a-safe-minimum-28-05-2014 (accessed 14 October 2021).

47. Ball J. Analysing the implementation and effects of safe staffing policies in acute hospitals. *Nurs Manage* 2020; 27: 35–40. https://doi.org/10.7748/nm.2020.e1904.

48. McClure ML, Poulin MA, Sovie MD, Wandelt MA. *Magnet Hospitals: Attraction and Retention of Professional Nurses.* Kansas City, MO: American Academy of Nursing Task Force on Nursing Practice in Hospitals; 1983.

49. Twigg D, McCullough K. Nurse retention: a review of strategies to create and enhance positive practice environments in clinical settings. *Int J Nurs Stud* 2014; 51: 85–92. https://doi.org/10.1016/j.ijnurstu.2013.05.015.

50. Halter M, Pelone F, Boiko O, et al. Interventions to reduce adult nursing turnover: a systematic review of systematic reviews. *Open Nurs J* 2017; 11: 108–23. https://doi.org/10.2174/1874434601711010108.

51. Nursing and Midwifery Council. *The NMC Register.* London: NMC; 2017. www.nmc.org.uk/globalassets/sitedocuments/data-reports/the-nmc-register-30-september-2017.pdf (accessed 14 October 2021).

52. Aiken LH, Smith HL, Lake ET. Lower Medicare mortality among a set of hospitals known for good nursing care. *Med Care* 1994; 32: 771–87. https://doi.org/10.1097/00005650-199408000-00002.

53. Kelly LA, McHugh MD, Aiken LH. Nurse outcomes in Magnet® and non-Magnet hospitals. *J Nurs Adm* 2012; 42: S44–9. https://doi.org/10.1097/01.NNA.0000420394.18284.4f.

54. Jones K. The benefits of Magnet status for nurses, patients and organisations. *Nurs Times* 2017; 113: 28–31. www.nursingtimes.net/roles/nurse-managers/the-benefits-of-magnet-status-for-nurses-patients-and-organisations-30-10-2017 (accessed 14 October 2021).

55. Kramer M. The Magnet hospitals: excellence revisited. *J Nurs Adm* 1990; 20: 35–44. https://doi.org/10.1097/00005110-199009000-00009.

56. Kramer M, Schmalenberg C. Magnet hospitals part II: institutions of excellence. *J Nurs Adm* 1988; 18: 11–9. https://doi.org/10.1097/00005110-198802010-00005.

57. Kutney-Lee A, Stimpfel AW, Sloane DM, et al. Changes in patient and nurse outcomes associated with Magnet hospital recognition. *Med Care* 2015; 53: 550–7. https://doi.org/10.1097/MLR.0000000000000355.

58. McHugh MD, Rochman MF, Sloane DM, et al. Better nurse staffing and nurse work environments associated with increased survival of in-hospital cardiac arrest patients. *Med Care* 2016; 54: 74–80. https://doi.org/10.1097/MLR.0000000000000456.

59. Scott JG, Sochalski J, Aiken L. Review of Magnet hospital research: findings and implications for professional nursing practice. *J Nurs Adm* 1999; 29: 9–19. https://doi.org/10.1097/00005110-199901000-00003.

60. Willis GP. *Raising the Bar: Shape of Caring: A Review of the Future Education and Training of Registered Nurses and Care Assistants.* London: Health Education England; 2015. www.hee.nhs.uk/sites/default/files/documents/2348-Shape-of-caring-review-FINAL.pdf (accessed 14 October 2021).

61. Royal College of Nursing. *The Magnet Recognition Programme: A Discussion of Its Development, Success and Challenges for Adoption in the UK.* London: RCN; 2015. www.rcn.org.uk/about-us/our-influencing-work/policy-briefings/POL-0915 (accessed 14 October 2021).

62. Friese CR, Xia R, Ghaferi A, Birkmeyer JD, Banerjee M. Hospitals in 'Magnet' program show better patient outcomes on mortality measures compared to non-'Magnet' hospitals. *Health Aff* 2015; 34: 986–92. https://doi.org/10.1377/hlthaff.2014.0793.

63. Mitchell G. New European study overhauling hospitals for nurse well-being. *Nurs Times*; 24 February 2020. www.nursingtimes.net/news/hospital/exclusive-new-european-study-overhauling-hospitals-for-nurse-wellbeing-24-02-2020 (accessed 14 October 2021).

64. Maben J, Morrow E, Ball J, Robert G, Griffiths P. *High Quality Care Metrics for Nursing.* London: National Nursing Research Unit, King's College London; 2012. www.kcl.ac.uk/nmpc/research/nnru/publications/reports/high-quality-care-metrics-for-nursing–nov-2012.pdf (accessed 14 October 2021).

65. Toulany T, Shojania K. Measurement for improvement. In: Dixon-Woods M, Brown K, Marjanovic S, et al., editors. *Elements of Improving Quality and Safety in Healthcare.* Cambridge: Cambridge University Press; forthcoming.

66. Drennan J, Duffield C, Scott AP, et al. A protocol to measure the impact of intentional changes to nurse staffing and skill-mix in medical and surgical wards. *J Adv Nurs* 2018; 74: 2912–21. https://doi.org/10.1111/jan.13796.

67. Department of Health, Ireland. *Framework for Safe Nurse Staffing and Skill Mix in General and Specialist Medical and Surgical Care Settings in Adult Hospitals in Ireland 2018: Final Report and Recommendations by the Taskforce on Staffing and Skill Mix for Nursing*. Dublin: Department of Health; 2018. https://assets.gov.ie/10011/e1a93e955329405694bb7b16aea50b98.pdf (accessed 14 October 2021).

68. Zoutman DE, Ford BD. Quality improvement in hospitals: barriers and facilitators. *Int J Health Care Qual Assur* 2017; 30: 16–24. https://doi.org/10.1108/ijhcqa-12-2015-0144.

69. Dixon-Woods M. How to improve healthcare improvement – an essay by Mary Dixon-Woods. *BMJ* 2019; 367: l5514. https://doi.org/10.1136/bmj.l5514.

70. Morrow E, Robert G, Maben J. Exploring the nature and impact of leadership on the local implementation of The Productive Ward Releasing Time to Care™. *J Health Organ Manage* 2014; 28: 154–76. https://doi.org/10.1108/JHOM-04-2014-0064.

71. Needleman J, Hassmiller S. The role of nurses in improving hospital quality and efficiency: real-world results. *Health Aff* 2009; 28: w625–33. https://doi.org/10.1377/hlthaff.28.4.w625.

72. Dixon-Woods M, Martin GP. Does quality improvement improve quality? *Future Hosp J* 2016; 3: 191–4. www.repository.cam.ac.uk/handle/1810/260182 (accessed 14 October 2021).

73. Edmondson A. Psychological safety and learning behavior in work teams. *Adm Sci Q* 1999; 44: 350–83. https://doi.org/10.2307/2666999.

74. Fried BJ, Edmondson AC. Teams and team effectiveness in health services organizations. In: Burns LR, Bradley EH, Weiner BJ, editors. *Shortell & Kaluzny's Health Care Management: Organization Design and Behavior*. 7th ed. Boston, MA: Cengage Learning; 2019: 98–131.

75. Frazier PA, Tix AP, Barron KE. "Testing moderator and mediator effects in counseling psychology research": correction to Frazier et al. *J Couns Psychol* 2004; 51: 157. https://doi.org/10.1037/0022-0167.51.2.157.

76. Newman A, Donohue R, Eva N. Psychological safety: a systematic review of the literature. *Hum Resour Manage* 2017; 27: 521–35. https://doi.org/10.1016/j.hrmr.2017.01.001.

77. Edmondson AC, Lei Z. Psychological safety: the history, renaissance, and future of an interpersonal construct. *Annu Rev Organ Psychol Organ Behav* 2014; 1: 23–43. https://doi.org/10.1146/annurev-orgpsych-031413-091305.

78. Goffman E. *Presentation of Self in Everyday Life*. Garden City, NY: Doubleday Anchor Books; 1959.

79. Schein EH, Bennis WG. *Personal and Organizational Change through Group Methods: The Laboratory Approach*. New York: Wiley; 1965.

80. Sanner B, Bunderson JS. When feeling safe isn't enough: contextualizing models of safety and learning in teams. *Organ Psychol Rev* 2015; 5: 224–43. https://doi.org/10.1177/2041386614565145.

81. Edmondson AC. Learning from mistakes is easier said than done: group and organizational influences on the detection and correction of human error. *J Appl Behav Sci* 1996; 32: 5–28. https://doi.org/10.1177/0021886396321001.

82. Edmondson AC, Roberto M, Tucker AL. *Children's Hospital and Clinics (A)*. Boston, MA: Harvard Business School (case 302-050); 2001, revised 2007. https://projects.iq.harvard.edu/files/sdpfellowship/files/childrens_hospital_and_clinics.pdf (accessed 9 December 2022).

83. Goodman JC, Villarreal P, Jones B. The social cost of adverse medical events, and what we can do about it. *Health Aff* 2011; 30: 590–5. https://doi.org/10.1377/hlthaff.2010.1256.

84. Reason J. Human error: models and management. *BMJ* 2000; 320: 768–70. https://doi.org/10.1136/bmj.320.7237.768.

85. Drury C. Coronavirus: NHS whistleblowers 'threatened with job loss' for speaking out on PPE. *The Independent*; 15 May 2020. www.independent.co.uk/news/uk/home-news/coronavirus-uk-nhs-ppe-whistleblowers-job-losses-ppe-a9515856.html (accessed 9 December 2022).

86. Dyer C. Covid-19: doctors are warned not to go public about PPE shortages. *BMJ* 2020; 369: m1592. https://doi.org/10.1136/bmj.m1592.

87. Mannion R, Davies H. Raising and responding to frontline concerns in healthcare. *BMJ* 2019; 366: l4944. https://doi.org/10.1136/bmj.l4944.

88. Jones A, Kelly D. Deafening silence? Time to reconsider whether organisations are silent or deaf when things go wrong. *BMJ Qual Saf* 2014; 23: 709–13. https://doi.org/10.1136/bmjqs-2013-002718.

89. Leroy H, Dierynck B, Anseel F, et al. Behavioral integrity for safety, priority of safety, psychological safety, and patient safety: a team-level study. *J Appl Psychol* 2012; 97: 1273–81. https://doi.org/10.1037/a0030076.

90. May DR, Gilson RL, Harter LM. The psychological conditions of meaningfulness, safety and availability and the engagement of the human spirit at work. *J Occup Organ Psychol* 2004; 77: 11–37. https://doi.org/10.1348/096317904322915892.

91. Chughtai AA, Buckley F. Exploring the impact of trust on research scientists' work engagement. *Pers Rev* 2013; 42: 396–421. https://doi.org/10.1108/PR-06-2011-0097.

92. Ulusoy N, Mölders C, Fischer S, et al. A matter of psychological safety: commitment and mental health in Turkish immigrant employees in Germany. *J Cross Cult Psychol* 2016; 47: 626–45. https://doi.org/10.1177/0022022115626513.

93. Rathert C, Ishqaidef G, May DR. Improving work environments in health care: test of a theoretical framework. *Health Care Manage Rev* 2009; 34: 334–43. https://doi.org/10.1097/HMR.0b013e3181abce2b.

94. Tucker AL, Nembhard IM, Edmondson AC. Implementing new practices: an empirical study of organizational learning in hospital intensive care units. *Manage Sci* 2007; 53: 894–907. https://doi.org/10.1287/mnsc.1060.0692.

95. Tucker AL, Edmondson AC. Why hospitals don't learn from failures: organizational and psychological dynamics that inhibit system change. *Calif Manage Rev* 2003; 45: 55–72. https://doi.org/10.2307/41166165.

96. Halbesleben JR, Rathert C. The role of continuous quality improvement and psychological safety in predicting work-arounds. *Health Care Manage Rev* 2008; 33: 134–44. https://doi.org/10.1097/01.Hmr.0000304505.04932.62.

97. Nembhard IM, Edmondson AC. Making it safe: the effects of leader inclusiveness and professional status on psychological safety and improvement efforts in health care teams. *J Organ Behav* 2006; 27: 941–66. https://doi.org/10.1002/job.413.

98. Liu S, Hu J, Li Y, Wang Z, Lin X. Examining the cross-level relationship between shared leadership and learning in teams: evidence from China. *Leadersh Q* 2014; 1: 282–95. https://doi.org/10.1016/j.leaqua.2013.08.006.

99. Edmondson AC, Bohmer RM, Pisano GP. Disrupted routines: team learning and new technology implementation in hospitals. *Adm Sci Q* 2001; 46: 685–716. https://doi.org/10.2307/3094828.

100. Fulop NJ, Ramsay AIG. Governance and leadership. In: Dixon-Woods M, Brown K, Marjanovic S, et al., editors. *Elements of Improving Quality and Safety in Healthcare*. Cambridge: Cambridge University Press; forthcoming.

101. Edmondson A. A safe harbor: social psychological factors effecting boundary spanning in work teams. In: Mannix B, Neale M, Wageman R, editors. *Research on Groups and Teams*. Greenwich, CT: JAI Press; 1999: 179–200.

102. Chen C, Liao J, Wen P. Why does formal mentoring matter? The mediating role of psychological safety and the moderating role of power distance orientation in the Chinese context. *Int J Hum Resour Manag* 2014; 25: 1112–30. https://doi.org/10.1080/09585192.2013.816861.

103. Singh B, Winkel DE, Selvarajan TT. Managing diversity at work: does psychological safety hold the key to racial differences in employee performance? *J Occup Organ Psychol* 2013; 86: 242–63. https://doi.org/10.1111/joop.12015.

104. Carmeli A, Gittell JH. High-quality relationships, psychological safety, and learning from failures in work organizations. *J Organ Behav* 2009; 30: 709–29. https://doi.org/10.1002/job.565.

105. Cross R, Edmondson AC, Murphy W. A noble purpose won't transform your company: leadership behaviors that nurture interpersonal collaboration are the true drivers of change. *Sloan Manage Rev* 2020; 61: 37–43. https://sloanreview.mit.edu/article/a-noble-purpose-alone-wont-transform-your-company (accessed 14 October 2021).

106. Roberto MA. Lessons from Everest: the interaction of cognitive bias, psychological safety, and system complexity. *Calif Manage Rev* 2002; 45: 136–58. https://doi.org/10.2307/41166157.

107. Ericksen J, Dyer L. Right from the start: exploring the effects of early team events on subsequent project team development and performance. *Adm Sci Q* 2004; 49: 438–71. https://doi.org/10.2307/4131442.

108. Edmondson AC. *The Fearless Organization: Creating Psychological Safety in the Workplace for Learning, Innovation, and Growth.* Hoboken, NJ: John Wiley; 2018.

109. World Health Organization. *Global Strategy on Human Resources for Health: Workforce 2030.* Geneva: WHO; 2016. www.who.int/hrh/resources/global_strategy_workforce2030_14_print.pdf (accessed 14 October 2021).

110. Bodenheimer T, Chen E, Bennett HD. Confronting the growing burden of chronic disease: can the U.S. health care workforce do the job? *Health Aff (Millwood)* 2009; 28: 64–74. https://doi.org/10.1377/hlthaff.28.1.64.

111. Health Education England. *NHS Staff and Learners' Mental Wellbeing Commission.* Birmingham: HEE; 2019. www.hee.nhs.uk/sites/default/files/documents/NHS%20%28HEE%29%20-%20Mental%20Wellbeing%20Commission%20Report.pdf (accessed 14 April 2022).

112. Boorman S. *Health and Well-Being: Final Report.* London: Department of Health; 2009. https://webarchive.nationalarchives.gov.uk/ukgwa/20130103004910/http://www.dh.gov.uk/en/Publicationsandstatistics/Publications/PublicationsPolicyAndGuidance/DH_108799 (accessed 14 October 2021).

113. British Medical Association. *Supporting Health and Wellbeing at Work.* London: BMA; 2018. www.bma.org.uk/media/2076/bma-supporting-health-and-wellbeing-at-work-oct-2018.pdf (accessed 14 April 2022).

114. Harvey SB, Laird B, Henderson M, Hotopf M. *The Mental Health of Health Care Professionals: A Review for the Department of Health.* London: National Clinic Assessment Service; 2009. https://webarchive.natio nalarchives.gov.uk/ukgwa/20130123201334/http://www.dh.gov.uk/en/ Publicationsandstatistics/Publications/PublicationsPolicyAndGuidance/ DH_113540 (accessed 12 April 2022).

115. Maben J, Latter S, Clark JM. The sustainability of ideals, values and the nursing mandate: evidence from a longitudinal qualitative study. *Nurs Inq* 2007; 14: 99–113. https://doi.org/10.1111/j.1440-1800.2007.00357.x.

116. Rupert PA, Miller AO, Dorociak KE. Preventing burnout: what does the research tell us? *Prof Psychol: Res Pract* 2015; 46: 168–74. https://doi .org/10.1037/a0039297.

117. Ham C. UK government's autumn statement: no relief for NHS and social care in England. *BMJ* 2016; 355: i6382. https://doi.org/10.1136/bmj.i6382.

118. Brand SL, Thompson Coon J, Fleming LE, et al. Whole-system approaches to improving the health and wellbeing of healthcare workers: a systematic review. *PLoS One* 2017; 12: e0188418. https://doi.org/ 10.1371/journal.pone.0188418.

119. Brooks SK, Gerada C, Chalder T. Review of literature on the mental health of doctors: are specialist services needed? *J Ment Health* 2011; 20: 146–56. https://doi.org/10.3109/09638237.2010.541300.

120. Afolabi A, Fernando S, Bottiglieri T. The effect of organisational factors in motivating healthcare employees: a systematic review. *Br J Healthcare Manage* 2018; 24: 603–10. https://doi.org/10.12968/bjhc.2018.24.12.603.

121. Demerouti E, Bakker AB, Nachreiner F, Schaufeli WB. The job demands-resources model of burnout. *J Appl Psychol* 2001; 86: 499–512. https://doi.org/10.1037/0021-9010.86.3.499.

122. Bakker AB, Demerouti E. The job demands-resources model: state of the art. *J Manage Psychol* 2007; 22: 309–28. https://doi.org/10.1108/ 02683940710733115.

123. Maben J, Peccei R, Adams M, et al. *Exploring the Relationship between Patients' Experiences of Care and the Influence of Staff Motivation, Affect and Wellbeing: Final Report.* London: NIHR Service Delivery and Organisation Programme; 2012. www.journalslibrary.nihr.ac.uk/ programmes/hsdr/081819213/# (accessed 14 October 2021).

124. Taylor C, Xyrichis A, Leamy MC, Reynolds E, Maben J. Can Schwartz Center Rounds support healthcare staff with emotional challenges at work, and how do they compare with other interventions aimed at providing similar support? A systematic review and scoping reviews. *BMJ Open* 2018; 8: e024254. https://doi.org/10.1136/bmjopen-2018-024254.

125. Sturgess J, Poulsen A. The prevalence of burnout in occupational therapists. *Occup Ther Ment Health* 1983; 3: 47–60. https://doi.org/10.1300/J004v03n04_05.

126. McCray LW, Cronholm PF, Bogner HR, Gallo JJ, Neill RA. Resident physician burnout: is there hope? *Fam Med* 2008; 40: 626–32. https://fammedarchives.blob.core.windows.net/imagesandpdfs/fmhub/fm2008/October/Laura626.pdf (accessed 14 October 2021).

127. Limb M. Stress levels of NHS staff are "astonishingly high" and need treating as a public health problem, says King's Fund. *BMJ* 2015; 351: h6003. https://doi.org/10.1136/bmj.h6003.

128. Select Committee on the Long-Term Sustainability of the NHS. *The Long-Term Sustainability of the NHS and Adult Social Care*. London: House of Lords; 2017. https://publications.parliament.uk/pa/ld201617/ldselect/ldnhssus/151/151.pdf (accessed 14 April 2022).

129. Stevenson D, Farmer P. *Thriving at Work: The Stevenson/Farmer Review of Mental Health and Employers*. London: Department for Work and Pensions, Department of Health and Social Care; 2017. www.gov.uk/government/publications/thriving-at-work-a-review-of-mental-health-and-employers (accessed 14 April 2022).

130. Dall'Ora C, Griffiths P, Ball J, Simon M, Aiken LH. Association of 12 h shifts and nurses' job satisfaction, burnout and intention to leave: findings from a cross-sectional study of 12 European countries. *BMJ Open* 2015; 5: e008331. https://doi.org/10.1136/bmjopen-2015-008331.

131. Hospital Consultants and Specialists Association. Who Cares for the Carers? HCSA Hospital Doctors' Stress Survey Reveals Shocking Results. *HCSA*; 11 September 2015. www.hcsa.com/news-views/news/2015/09/stress-survey-initial.aspx (accessed 14 April 2022).

132. Van der Heijden B, Brown Mahoney C, Xu Y. Impact of job demands and resources on nurses' burnout and occupational turnover intention towards an age-moderated mediation model for the nursing profession. *Int J Environ Res Public Health* 2019; 16: 2011. https://doi.org/10.3390/ijerph16112011.

133. Willard-Grace R, Knox M, Huang B, et al. Burnout and health care workforce turnover. *Ann Fam Med* 2019; 17: 36–41. https://doi.org/10.1370/afm.2338.

134. Hall LH, Johnson J, Watt I, Tsipa A, O'Connor DB. Healthcare staff wellbeing, burnout, and patient safety: a systematic review. *PLoS One* 2016; 11: e0159015. https://doi.org/10.1371/journal.pone.0159015.

135. Raleigh VS, Hussey D, Seccombe I, Qi R. Do associations between staff and inpatient feedback have the potential for improving patient

experience? An analysis of surveys in NHS acute trusts in England. *BMJ Qual Saf* 2009; 18: 347–54. https://doi.org/10.1136/qshc.2008 .028910.

136. Edwards N. *Lost in Translation: Why Are Patients More Satisfied with the NHS Than the Public?* London: The NHS Confederation; 2006. www .ipsos.com/sites/default/files/migrations/en-uk/files/Assets/Docs/ Archive/Polls/nhs-confederation.pdf (accessed 12 April 2022).

137. Aiken LH, Clarke SP, Sloane DM, Sochalski J, Silber JH. Hospital nurse staffing and patient mortality, nurse burnout, and job dissatisfaction. *JAMA* 2002; 288: 1987–93. https://doi.org/10.1001/jama.288.16.1987.

138. West E. Management matters: the link between hospital organisation and quality of patient care. *BMJ Qual Saf* 2001; 10: 40–8. https://doi.org/ 10.1136/qhc.10.1.40.

139. Adams A, Bond S. Hospital nurses' job satisfaction, individual and organizational characteristics. *J Adv Nurs* 2000; 32: 536–43. https://doi .org/10.1046/j.1365-2648.2000.01513.x.

140. Reeves S, Lewin S. Interprofessional collaboration in the hospital: strategies and meanings. *J Health Serv Res Policy* 2004; 9: 218–25. https://doi .org/10.1258/1355819042250140.

141. Carter A, West M. *Teams and Staff Commitment.* Aston: Aston Organisation Development Network; 1999.

142. Burnes B, Pope R. Negative behaviours in the workplace: a study of two primary care trusts in the NHS. *Int J Public Sect Manage* 2007; 20: 285–303. https://doi.org/10.1108/09513550710750011.

143. Bodenheimer T, Sinsky C. From triple to quadruple aim: care of the patient requires care of the provider. *Ann Fam Med* 2014; 12: 573–6. https://doi.org/10.1370/afm.1713.

144. Pezaro S, Clyne W, Fulton EA. A systematic mixed-methods review of interventions, outcomes and experiences for midwives and student midwives in work-related psychological distress. *Midwifery* 2017; 50: 163–73. https://doi.org/10.1016/j.midw.2017.04.003.

145. Irving JA, Dobkin PL, Park J. Cultivating mindfulness in health care professionals: a review of empirical studies of mindfulness-based stress reduction (MBSR). *Complement Ther Clin Pract* 2009; 15: 61–6. https:// doi.org/10.1016/j.ctcp.2009.01.002.

146. Burton A, Burgess C, Dean S, Koutsopoulou GZ, Hugh-Jones S. How effective are mindfulness-based interventions for reducing stress among healthcare professionals? A systematic review and meta-analysis. *Stress Health* 2017; 33: 3–13. https://doi.org/10.1002/smi.2673.

147. Lomas T, Medina JC, Ivtzan I, Rupprecht S, Eiroa-Orosa FJ. A systematic review of the impact of mindfulness on the well-being of healthcare professionals. *J Clin Psychol* 2018; 74: 319–55. https://doi.org/10.1002/jclp.22515.

148. Wheeler S, Richards K. *The Impact of Clinical Supervision on Counsellors and Therapists, Their Practice and Their Clients: A Systematic Review of the Literature.* Lutterworth: British Association for Counselling and Psychotherapy; 2007. www.bacp.co.uk/events-and-resources/research/publications/impact-of-clinical-supervision-on-counsellors-and-therapists-their-practice-and-their-clients (accessed 12 April 2022).

149. White E, Winstanley J. Clinical supervision for mental health professionals: the evidence base. *Soc Work Soc Sci Rev* 2011; 1493: 77–94. https://journals.whitingbirch.net/index.php/SWSSR/article/view/502 (accessed 12 April 2022).

150. Wallbank S. Maintaining professional resilience through group restorative supervision. *Community Pract* 2013; 86: 26–8. www.researchgate.net/publication/256288337_Maintaining_professional_resilience_through_group_restorative_supervision (accessed 14 October 2021).

151. Maben J, Bridges J. Covid-19: supporting nurses' psychological and mental health. *J Clin Nurs* 2020; 29: 2742–50. https://doi.org/10.1111/jocn.15307.

152. Pipe TB, Buchda VL, Launder S, et al. Building personal and professional resources of resilience and agility in the healthcare workplace. *Stress Health* 2012; 28: 11–22. https://doi.org/10.1002/smi.1396.

153. Foster K, Cuzzillo C, Furness T. Strengthening mental health nurses' resilience through a workplace resilience programme: a qualitative inquiry. *J Psychiatr Ment Health Nurs* 2018; 25: 338–48. https://doi.org/10.1111/jpm.12467.

154. Traynor M. Guest editorial: what's wrong with resilience. *J Res Nurs* 2018; 23: 5–8. https://doi.org/10.1177/1744987117751458.

155. Carrieri D, Mattick K, Pearson M, et al. Optimising strategies to address mental ill-health in doctors and medical students: 'Care Under Pressure' realist review and implementation guidance. *BMC Med* 2020; 18: 76. https://doi.org/10.1186/s12916-020-01532-x.

156. Awa WL, Plaumann M, Walter U. Burnout prevention: a review of intervention programs. *Patient Educ Couns* 2010; 78: 184–90. https://doi.org/10.1016/j.pec.2009.04.008.

157. Sikka R, Morath JM, Leape L. The quadruple aim: care, health, cost and meaning in work. *BMJ Qual Saf* 2015; 24: 608–10. https://doi.org/10.1136/bmjqs-2015-004160.

158. Maben J, Taylor C, Dawson J, et al. A realist informed mixed-methods evaluation of Schwartz Center Rounds® in England. *Health Serv Deliv Res* 2018; 6: 37. https://doi.org/10.3310/hsdr06370.

159. McCarthy I, Taylor C, Leamy M, Reynolds E, Maben J. 'We needed to talk about it': the experience of sharing the emotional impact of health care work as a panellist in Schwartz Center Rounds® in the UK. *J Health Serv Res Policy* 2020; 26: 20–7. https://doi.org/10.1177/1355819620925512.

160. NHS England, NHS Improvement. *Interim NHS People Plan*. London: NHS; 2019. www.longtermplan.nhs.uk/wp-content/uploads/2019/05/Interim-NHS-People-Plan_June2019.pdf (accessed 14 April 2022).

161. Dixon-Woods M, McNicol S, Martin G. Ten challenges in improving quality in healthcare: lessons from the Health Foundation's programme evaluations and relevant literature. *BMJ Qual Saf* 2012; 21: 876–84. https://doi.org/10.1136/bmjqs-2011-000760.

162. Detert JR, Burris ER. Leadership behavior and employee voice: is the door really open? *Acad Manage J* 2007; 50: 869–84. https://doi.org/10.5465/AMJ.2007.26279183.

163. Barzallo Salazar MJ, Minkoff H, Bayya J, et al. Influence of surgeon behavior on trainee willingness to speak up: a randomized controlled trial. *J Am Coll Surg* 2014; 219: 1001–7. www.sciencedirect.com/science/article/abs/pii/S1072751514014690 (accessed 12 April 2022).

164. Riskin A, Erez A, Foulk TA, et al. Rudeness and medical team performance. *Pediatrics* 2017; 139: e20162305. https://doi.org/10.1542/peds.2016-2305.

165. Nembhard IM, Tucker AL. Deliberate learning to improve performance in dynamic service settings: evidence from hospital intensive care units. *Organ Sci* 2011; 22: 907–22. https://doi.org/10.1287/orsc.1100.0570.

166. Maben J, King A. Engaging NHS staff in research. *BMJ* 2019; 365: l4040. https://doi.org/10.1136/bmj.l4040.

167. Mannion R. Making culture change happen. In: Dixon-Woods M, Brown K, Marjanovic S, et al., editors. *Elements of Improving Quality and Safety in Healthcare*. Cambridge: Cambridge University Press; 2022. https://doi.org/10.1017/9781009236935.

168. Ball J. Special collection editorial: 'Enough Nurses?'. *J Res Nurs* 2017; 22: 566–71. https://doi.org/10.1177/1744987117740421.

169. National Institute for Health Research. *Staffing on Wards: Making Decisions about Healthcare Staffing, Improving Effectiveness and*

Supporting Staff to Care Well. NIHR Dissemination Centre; 2019. https://doi.org/10.3310/themedreview-03553.

170. Edmondson AC. *Teaming: How Organizations Learn, Innovate and Compete in the Knowledge Economy*. San Francisco, CA: Jossey-Bass; 2012.
171. Burns L, Bradley E, Weiner B, editors. *Shortell & Kaluzny's Health Care Management: Organization Design and Behavior*. 7th ed. Boston, MA: Cengage Learning; 2019.

Cambridge Elements ≡

Improving Quality and Safety in Healthcare

Editors-in-Chief
Mary Dixon-Woods
THIS Institute (The Healthcare Improvement Studies Institute)

Mary is Director of THIS Institute and is the Health Foundation Professor of Healthcare Improvement Studies in the Department of Public Health and Primary Care at the University of Cambridge. Mary leads a programme of research focused on healthcare improvement, healthcare ethics, and methodological innovation in studying healthcare.

Graham Martin
THIS Institute (The Healthcare Improvement Studies Institute)

Graham is Director of Research at THIS Institute, leading applied research programmes and contributing to the institute's strategy and development. His research interests are in the organisation and delivery of healthcare, and particularly the role of professionals, managers, and patients and the public in efforts at organisational change.

Executive Editor
Katrina Brown
THIS Institute (The Healthcare Improvement Studies Institute)

Katrina is Communications Manager at THIS Institute, providing editorial expertise to maximise the impact of THIS Institute's research findings. She managed the project to produce the series.

Editorial Team
Sonja Marjanovic
RAND Europe

Sonja is Director of RAND Europe's healthcare innovation, industry, and policy research. Her work provides decision-makers with evidence and insights to support innovation and improvement in healthcare systems, and to support the translation of innovation into societal benefits for healthcare services and population health.

Tom Ling
RAND Europe

Tom is Head of Evaluation at RAND Europe and President of the European Evaluation Society, leading evaluations and applied research focused on the key challenges facing health services. His current health portfolio includes evaluations of the innovation landscape, quality improvement, communities of practice, patient flow, and service transformation.

Ellen Perry
THIS Institute (The Healthcare Improvement Studies Institute)

Ellen supported the production of the series during 2020–21.

About the Series

The past decade has seen enormous growth in both activity and research on improvement in healthcare. This series offers a comprehensive and authoritative set of overviews of the different improvement approaches available, exploring the thinking behind them, examining evidence for each approach, and identifying areas of debate.

Improving Quality and Safety in Healthcare

Printed in the United States
by Baker & Taylor Publisher Services